"SMACKHEADS DON'T GET FAT"

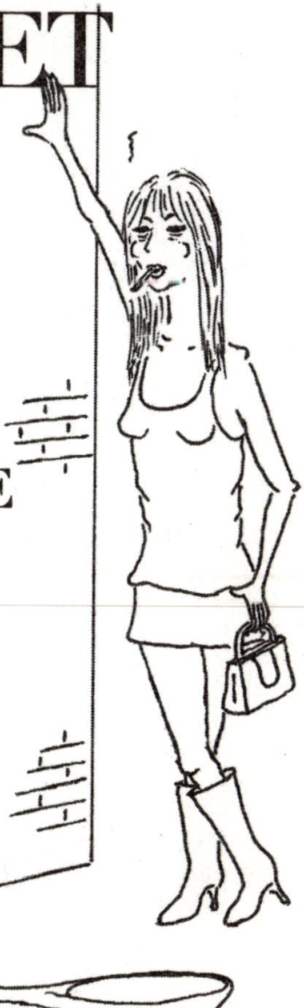

THE MORALLY QUESTIONABLE DIET BOOK

By
Dr. C. Harlatan
with Madame X

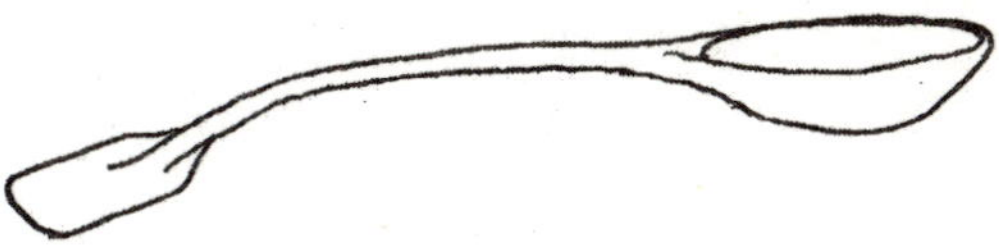

Crombie Jardine
PUBLISHING LIMITED
Office 2, 3 Edgar Buildings
George Street
Bath
BA1 2FJ
www.crombiejardine.com

Published by Crombie Jardine Publishing Limited
First edition, 2006

ISBN 13 digit: 978-1-905102-70-9

ISBN 10 digit: 1-905102-70-4

Cover illustration by Bob Gibbs
Design and some additional illustrations by www.glensaville.com
Printed and bound in Great Britain by
Cox and Wyman Ltd, Reading, Berks

ADVERTISSEMENT

TRES IMPORTANT

VERY IMPORTANT WARNING:

This book is meant to be FUNNY. The views and ideas contained herein clearly should not be adopted by ANYONE. If you are seriously tempted to actually try any of these diets then you are a MORON and the world will doubtless be a cleaner place after your inevitable early DEATH for which the authors and publisher accept no responsibility whatsoever.

Yes, you heard us, all the formulas and suggestions herein are DANGEROUS and we are hereby telling you not to attempt or to undertake any of them.

Finally, anything purporting to be a fact is either not true or not checked or both.

DO NOT ATTEMPT THESE DIETS!

'. . . any philosopher worthy of the name knows that, in itself, desire – unlike pleasure – is a source of suffering, pain and hatred.'

Michel Houellebecq, French novelist

CONTENTS

OUVERTURE

Alors, people ask me ''ow do you do it? 'ow come you are so lovely and slim? Is it because you are *française* and you buy all your food from the market of the farmers, never touch the convenience meals and only have one glass of *vin* with dinner?' I tell them '*Non!* I don't 'ave time for *le dîner*. I am busy *le soir!*' But I will tell you *mon secret*, and it is a thing that has long been known and discretely passed down through generations of women in my *milieu*. I am a *pute*, 'ow you say it, *une prostituée*, a lady of the night. I work very hard at my job and this is *why je ne suis pas grosse*.

I have also another *secret*. I am a user of certain chemicals that are *très intéressants*. And if there's *une chose* that is *certaine, mes petits choux,* it is that *les* Smackheads *do not get fat*.

Now, I must introduce you to Dr C Harlatan, a scientist of great renown and great thinness, with whom I have devised these diet plans. We have put together our invaluable knowledge and experience to bring you our diets *merveilleux*. He will explain all.

Bonne chance!

Madame X, Paris 2006

POURQUOI YOU NEED TO BE THIN

100% OF FAT PEOPLE DIE

POURQUOI TOUS LES AUTRES REGIMES SONT MERDE

WHY ALL THE OTHER DIETS ARE SHIT

If you've tried all the others – Atkins, GI, Cabbage Soup, being French, going to the South Beach, Detox, F-plan, to name but a few – and wondered why they don't work, or rather only work for a while before you put the pounds back on, this book, and specifically an *MQ* diet might be for you.

Literally minutes of research have revealed to us that the failure of the other diets is due to the BP factor. Let me show you how this works in a very scientific graph.

'NORMAL' DIET

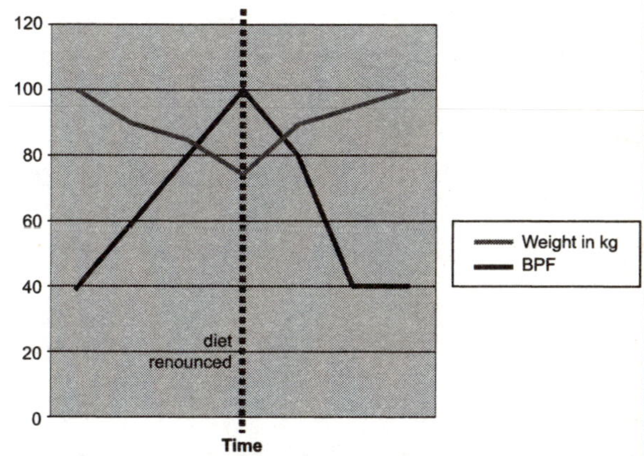

However this book will introduce you to the MQQ. The MQQ factor successfully counteracts the BPF. As a result you will keep going on your diet – probably for the rest of your life. And you know what? You won't even miss the food. This is why these diets work.

SO WHAT'S BPF AND MQQ?

BPF is the **B**oring **P**rig **F**actor.

MQQ is the **M**orally **Q**uestionable **Q**uotient.

The BPF is quite easy to spot in the dietee. You are having a BPF reaction when you refuse your lovely pasta dinner at a friend's house because you are on the Atkins. It is what you experience when you won't go to the pub while indulging in Detox. It's what happens when you can't eat a banana *because it contains the wrong fucking type of glucose*. You become quite an annoying person.

So the pounds drop off to start with, but take a look at the chart on page 11! As the pounds drop off your boring quotient goes through the roof. You might find that you get fewer dinner invitations. Friends no longer drop round. You realise that everyone at work has gone to the pub on a Friday afternoon, but 'forgotten' to ask you. A significant increase in BPF level normally means that you are forced to renounce your diet in order to *get a life*, at which point BPF immediately decreases, but you gain weight.

Research has shown that MQQ (morally questionable quotient) actually fights BPF in your brain. The result? You stay on your diet for longer. So if you want to shed weight and keep it shed you really should try a morally questionable diet.

HOW MQQ WORKS

Just like other diets MQQ requires you to embrace a committed lifestyle choice. However, because what you are doing is morally questionable you are less likely to get bored and give up. Think about it. It is hard to be a boring prig when you are quaffing a large bottle of wine or shooting up.

Specific aspects of the MQQ diet you choose will inhibit appetite too. This works on a number of levels. For example, food doesn't tend to be the first thing on your mind when waiting for your next solvent fix. Your new lifestyle will *distract* you beautifully. And, depending on the diet you choose, your appetite may be inhibited chemically as well as psychologically.

And, as we shall see, many of the diets presented here also work to contain the almost inevitable weight gain associated with middle and old age by ACTIVELY WORKING TO REDUCE LIFE EXPECTANCY.

What is more, Madame X and I know that with food and lifestyle one size very much does not suit all. The great thing about MQQ is that there are many different diet plans to choose from. All you need to do is find the one that suits you. If the first one you try doesn't work don't panic.

Just pick another! Before long you will find one that suits you. And will you have fun along the way? You bet!

Madame X comments

I like to talk about the *frisson* that the morally questionable diet can give you. Very French, *très élégant, n'est-ce pas?* Poor Monsieur Atkins. He never had that *joie*.

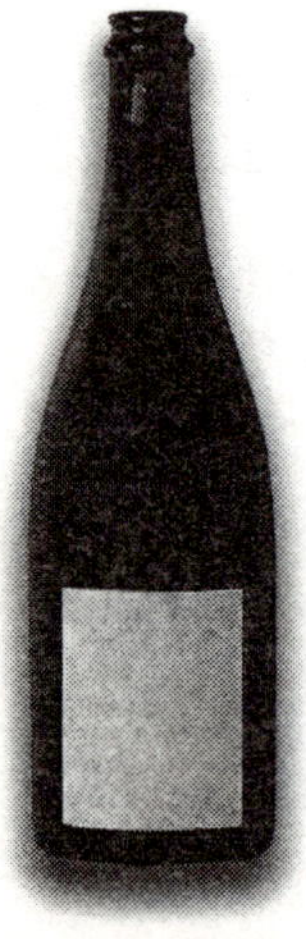

CHOOSING THE RIGHT MQQ DIET FOR YOU

The fun begins here where you get to choose the right diet plan for you. Everyone is different so what might work for you might be totally different to what would work for others. The trick is to find a diet that you are comfortable with and what is suited to your personality and situation in life.

Confused?

To start you off it might help to ask yourself the following questions:

- **How old am I?** If very young you might have problems of access or income. Perhaps try glue sniffing or why not make the most of your natural youthful narcissism? If approaching the autumn of your spell on earth have you considered anorexia? The Jain religion, for example, finds this a wonderfully spiritual way to grow dead gracefully.

- **Am I a man or a lady?** Research has shown that heartbreak works well for the guys but not for the girls. If a lady you could try adultery... or why not hunger striking?

- **How do I feel about breaking the law?** No problem if you don't fancy it! Just steer clear of the Class A drug diet regimes of smack and speed. Perhaps good old-fashioned alcoholism or chain smoking might be the way to go.

- **Do I like travel?** Well it'll be no surprise to you that we feel the Residents of a War-Torn Territory diet might be the one for you. If you prefer the sedentary lifestyle then don't worry! Most of the other diets can be done from the comfort of your own home[1].

- **Do I want to meet others?** Being a prostitute is a great way to break the ice.

Still confused? Do all of the diets appeal? This is the time to embark on our…

[1] For as long as you can pay the mortgage or rent in the case of some diets in this book.

WHICH DIET IS RIGHT FOR YOU FLOW CHART

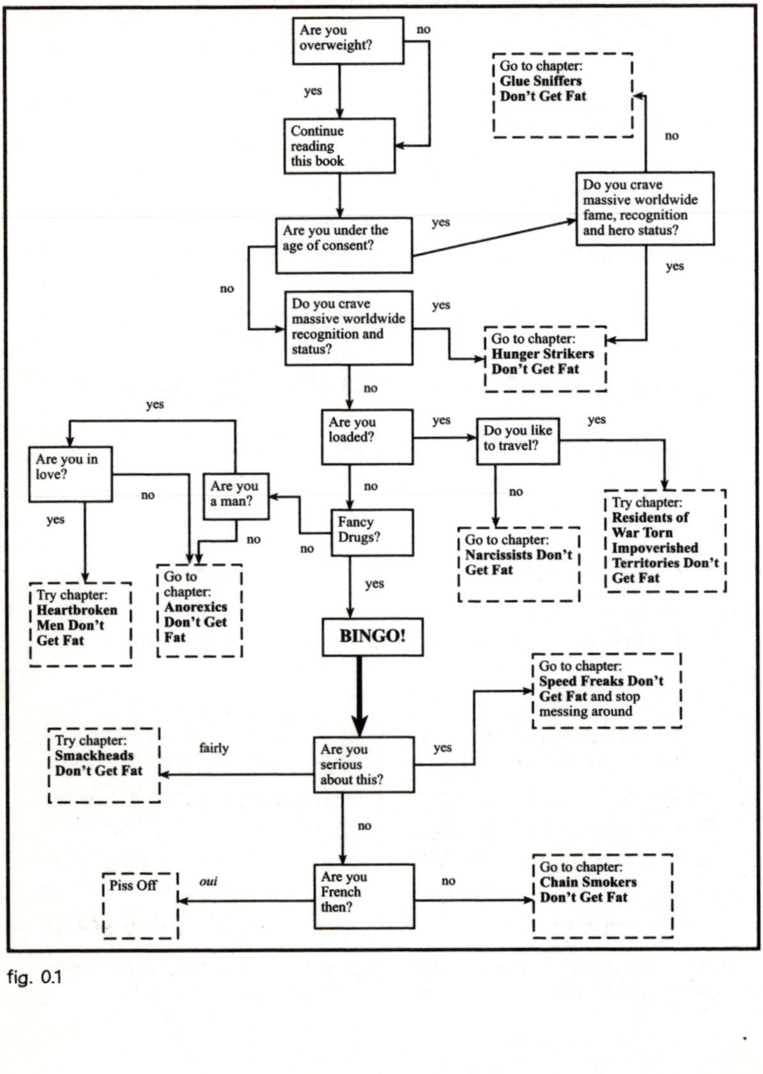

fig. 0.1

You don't even have to do one diet at a time. You could try combination diets. The Venn diagram below can help you compare criteria.

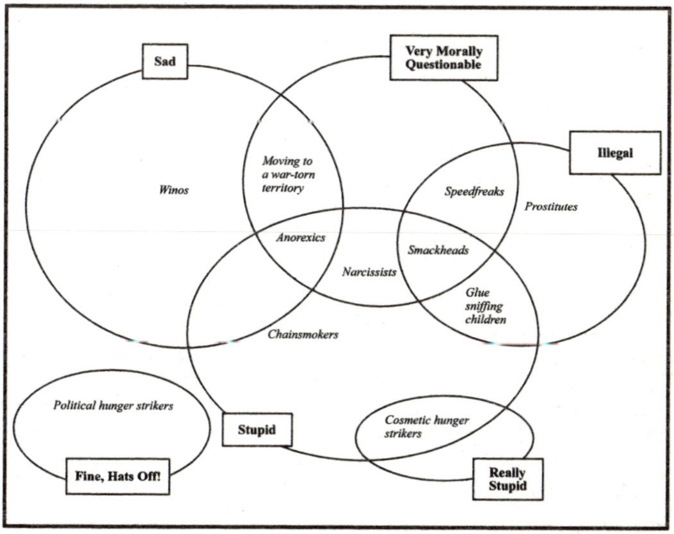

fig. 0.2

Are you confused as to whether something is morally questionable? Perhaps you think we've got it wrong here. Well, one of the tricky things about morality is that it is relative. Where some people think that being a prostitute is sinful, others think it is fine so long as no one is getting hurt. While some baulk at telling white lies, other people think that telling huge political whoppers on the international arena is just fine and dandy.

At the end of every section we'll tell you what other diets the chosen plan will work well with, and, just as crucially, the ones that don't mix. Enjoy your diet Mix 'n' Match – just look for the box at the end of every chapter! Like this:

DIET MIX 'N' MATCH DIET MIX 'N' MATCH DIET MIX 'N' MATCH DIET MI

You can combine this diet with...

Avoid...

SMACKHEADS DON'T GET FAT

Sometimes the most obvious things are the hardest to see. If you really want to lose weight – and for that weight to stay lost – you really should consider mainlining Street Quality heroin.

Don't be put off by issues of cost, accessibility and legality for, as we shall see, all these factors are very easily dealt with and can, in themselves, be beneficial to our cause. And don't be put off either by prejudices or needle-phobia – if you're really determined to lose weight it is worth persevering through the first few days; and that, indeed, is all it takes, for (and here is the real beauty and genius of this plan) the intrinsic highly-addictive nature of heroin, gear, smack, junk or horse makes sticking to the regime a doddle once those initial qualms have been overcome. You will find that your insatiable hunger for this magical wonder stuff will override all those issues you first had. Brilliant, eh?

Golden Brown indeed.

Fact: Tests indicate that people who use skag think about food 90% less than those not on skag.

WHY IT WORKS

The key to the success of the heroin-dependent diet revolves around one vital factor: self-worth. It is the destruction of this which is fundamental to your achieving your goals. But, again, don't be daunted if this sounds difficult – as fig. 1.1 clearly shows, as time progresses and your heroin intake increases, your self-worth will naturally fall away. Trust me on this one.

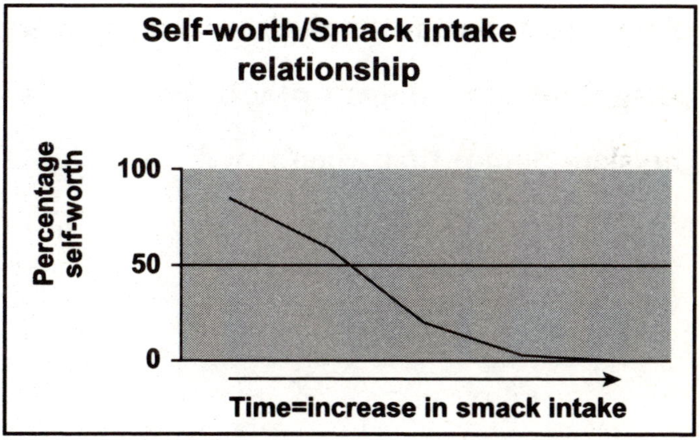

fig. 1.1

Before long, as you can see, your self-worth quotient will reach the magic zero and the ONLY THING in the world that will matter will be your next fix and you'll be ready to watch those pounds simply fall away.

It is obvious, I hope, that by the time this stage is reached, food will be pretty much the last thing on your mind. You will of course from time to time find yourself wanting or needing to eat and you should in no way be worried about that. It is another of the great beauties and advantages of this plan over so many others (even some in this very book!) that when you feel the desire for food you can eat as much as you want of whatever you want!

And here's why – it's yet another magical quality of our hypodermic miracle worker. You will naturally find that the food types that you crave, once you've become fully accustomed to the programme, will have VIRTUALLY NO nutritional value whatsoever! Ice cream. Chips. Fish fingers. Easy, convenient, pre-packaged rubbish to which you will give no thought, barely taste and sicken of almost instantly. You might even actually be sick and purge your body of whatever small amounts of goodness you have ingested.

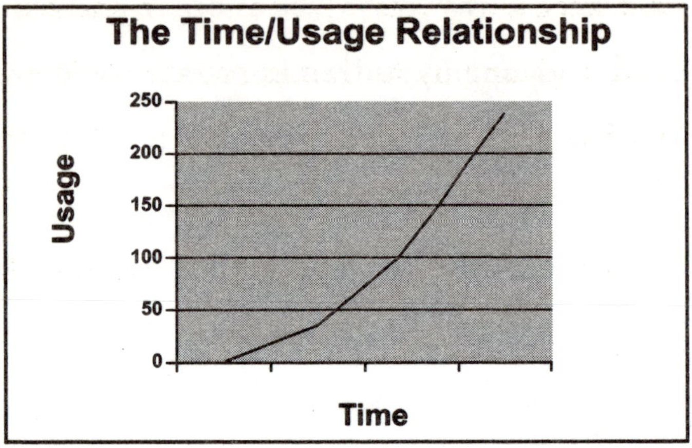

fig. 1.2

Another factor which makes the junk plan so successful is the ease with which usage naturally increases. Again don't be daunted – you will have to make NO EFFORT WHATSOEVER to achieve the vastly increased consumption which will put you on to the next stage of rapid weight loss. Once your body has become totally addicted to heroin you will find that you quite simply have no choice. How this is actually sustained we will come to later in the chapter, but rest assured you will be as drawn and gaunt and, goddammit, as thin as anyone could ever wish to be.

You will, in fact, to all intents and purposes, be BARELY ALIVE.

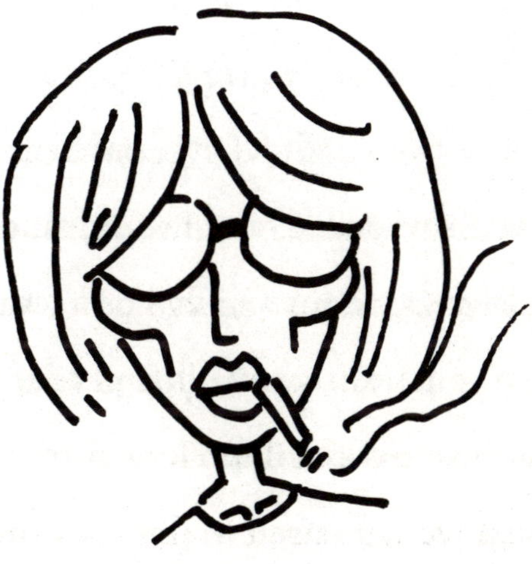

GETTING STARTED

Finding a dealer

'But I have no idea where I would get hold of a bunch of heroin.'

Rubbish.

Fact: every town has a heroin scene. You just need to know where to look. And if you live in a tiny hamlet or village you're just going to have to get on a bus. (You could drive, but bear in mind driving while whacked out of your mind on junk is extremely hazardous and you don't want to die a fatty, do you?) Also, once you get further into the programme you will no longer own a car so you may as well get used to life without it.

Okay. So, we're in our town or city. Most of us will know where to go. The 'rough' area – it's not rocket science. If you really don't know where the rough part of your town is you can always ask – try a passer-by or tourist information. Pretend to be a visitor who wants to avoid the places that are 'unsafe at night'. Because that, dear future-waif, is where you are going.

Depending on the type of town you're in your strategy will vary slightly, although some rules work for all cases.

- Wait until after dark. Obviously. If you're lucky you may find your man waiting for you at the corner; you may even get approached by him since...

- you have, again obviously, dressed in something extremely 'street'. Over casual. No suits or dresses.

- And remember: think like a junkie, walk like a junkie and your path to actually becoming one will be a lot smoother and shorter.

- Look like you're looking. Loiter. Look shifty. Dart your eyes.

And soon, sure enough, you will either be approached or you will see that shadowy figure (acting a little like you) whom you can edgily wander over to and ask: 'Got anything?' Don't be afraid. This is the first step towards a new you. Seize the moment.

If you find yourself in a town with no street scene you will have to venture into a bar. Keep your eyes peeled for the sunken eyes, high cheekbones and washboard stomach of the truly dedicated. Don't be intimidated by this image of perfection: it will soon be you!

Another trick is to break the first rule and hit the area and its hostelries at midday. All those putting away super-strength lager at lunchtime will doubtless know where to send you, even if they're not actually smackheads themselves.

Your First Hit

'But I wouldn't know what to do with it even if I managed to get hold of some.'

Okay, so we'll go with the premise that you have no initiative and have never seen *Trainspotting*. It's time to learn one very important and basic fact that will form the root of your existence for the rest of your life: **a junkie will do pretty much anything for a hit and *absolutely* anything for a free one.** So ask and cajole.

When you've found your supply ask where you can go and sort yourself out. Say you can sort him out something too and he'll lead you straight to his place – his flat possibly, a disused garage or similar more probably. Ask him to help fix it for you; say you've always done it with friends. Do *not* say it's your first time. Getting mugged is no fun. But remember, in some way this man is, temporarily, your best friend: you're paying; he loves you. In another, more accurate, way he is absolutely *not* your friend. Do not have huge quantities of cash or credit cards about your person – you're about to mong out in a squalid and filthy back street with a complete stranger who also happens to be a desperate junkie. But apart from that, put yourself squarely in this man's hands.

He is your future.

Let it be known that you are around to stay and will back the next day for more because:

- This is true and he's more likely to be around if he has a definite sale arranged.

- He's less likely to smash your skull open for your loose change and bus pass.

Last, but most important of all, remember that sharing[1] needles is a sign of good manners and trust. And besides, you didn't bring your own, did you?

It's worth noting that at this point you may feel unbelievably euphoric. Life might seem better than sex. You could just be at the single most fantastic moment of your life. Do not worry. Do not panic. And make no rash plans. This is a stage that has to be gone through – it is short lived and will never, ever return. Within a week this dangerous and potentially fattening *joie de vivre* will be replaced by sullen edginess and self-loathing and the last thing you'll feel like is rewarding yourself with a good square meal. Stay strong.

[1] Publisher's note: extremely dangerous – don't do it!

ACTION PLAN

Well, you've taken the first step and deserve a pat on the back. DON'T GIVE YOURSELF ONE. Remember what we said about self-worth?

Well here's the **Self-Worth Cycle of Fatness**:

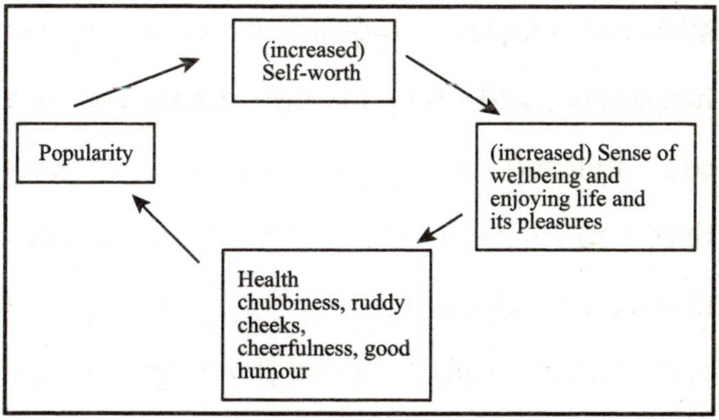

fig. 1.3

After two or three circuits you will find that you've turned into a fucking whale. Beware!

So when you get home after your first night of getting mashed off your face and rolling around in your own filth – stay focused! No food. No nothing. Just focus on that sense of infinite wellbeing and happiness that you felt. That way you'll be sure to go back again tonight. As I say, this will not last. It's just nature's crazy way of getting us through this difficult non-addicted opening phase. Once you've become heroin dependent it is no longer necessary for it to be a pleasant experience since there's no way in hell you'll ever kick it. *The human body really is truly miraculous.*

One of the main benefits of the skag diet is the brevity of the action plan and the relatively low levels of action or planning involved. Many diets have a twelve-week plan before you are accustomised enough to have any hope of sticking with it. With this programme, on the other hand, lasting results can be obtained *in just four days*! However, we will be working here on a timescale of one week to radically and permanently change your life for the thinner.

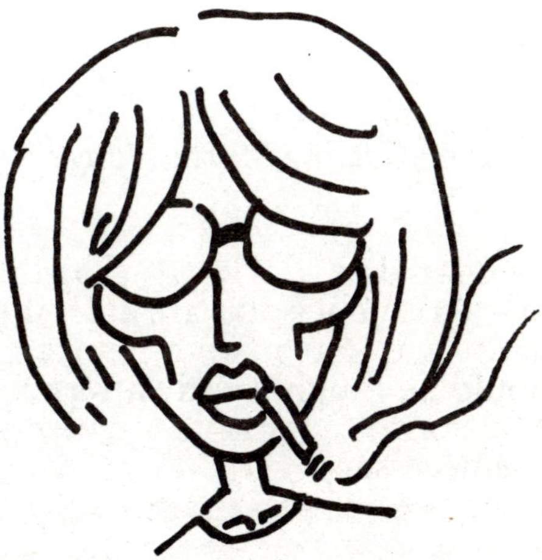

YOUR SEVEN-DAY MIRACLE PLAN

It is to be noted that your day will now be structured in a different way to the manner in which you have become accustomed. A successful and slender smackhead's day will never start before noon and usually begins far later than that.

So…

Day One – See *Getting Started (page 30).*

Day Two – Arise once you are able, if not later – this should be roughly early afternoon. Food will not be necessary.

At this delicate stage of your journey contact with the outside world, at least the outside world as you used to know it, is very much to be discouraged. It can only lead to a weakening of your resolve or the persistent self-interested attempts by so-called friends to lure you back to the world of tubby indulgence which you are now working so hard to put behind you.

So I would strongly advise a pre-emptive strike. Many have succeeded in this plan by simply refusing to answer the door or the telephone throughout this tricky opening period. For those of us who are sadly not so strong, I would recommend a few cleansing phone calls as follows:

Family and friends: 'I'm going away for a while – don't worry, I'm fine but I just need a bit of time to myself.' (Both of which, incidentally, are true.)

Work: 'I quit.'

So you can now disconnect the phone and the doorbell safe in the knowledge that by the time anyone properly worries and tries to find you, you will no longer care in the slightest about the truth, them, or indeed pretty much anything at all. It may well be the case that by the time they do try to make contact you will no longer be living at your current address anyway.

The rest of the day should be taken up with gentle televisual entertainment and as little physical activity as possible. Remember, exercise will only encourage the development of unsightly muscle – throughout this programme the aim with any weight that is retained is that it should hang as close to the bone as possible and not form itself into unsightly artificially toned bulges.

Hunger *will* strike. Again, do NOT panic yourself into eating, for I will now let you into a priceless and timeless secret of the H-lover:

Beer.

At this early stage, any time you feel a hunger pang, simply substitute a snack with a beer. Nothing too strong for now (plenty of time for that later), just enough to fill you up a little and produce a mild sense of wellbeing. Although you may have been told by other so-called diets that beer is fattening, you will soon find that when used as a central part of a heroin-based regime it works wonderfully as a suppressant of appetite, self-worth and, most crucially, lucidity between fixes.

Soon you will find it is time for your nocturnal *rendez-vous*. By now, hopefully, you will have a few leads – ideally the same supplier as last night. If not, simply repeat the procedure outlined in *Getting Started*. If your man is not where you expected, do not be discouraged – remember the seminal work of Lou Reed and his (timeless) advice that 'the first thing that you learn is that you've always got to wait.' Something will come through for you. It always does.

Besides, shivering nervously on a street corner never plumped anyone up for Christmas!

Day Three – An intermediate day. Often a dangerous one. If you didn't make those calls and disconnect those 'avenues of weakness' DO IT NOW. Draw the curtains. Keep drinking the beer. Keep the television on. As with hunger, if you find yourself experiencing boredom don't panic. This, as with every other emotion and sensation, will, in time, fade to virtually nothing. Remember *only a truly empty mind will allow room for truly sunken cheeks.* Boredom is merely a sign that you still have a little way to go – it will pass.

On tonight's trip downtown, you should be ready for the next step, although if you're not quite ready, or get unlucky, simply repeat Day Two until conditions are right. Hopefully by now you should be in a position where you have enough experience to fix yourself up, so on tonight's trip we're going to buy ourselves a little supply, enough possibly to last for a day or two. This will be good practice although in no way represents your future. At this stage you have a disposable income that will soon seem like a whole other world. Hand to Mouth, the real slimmer's friend, is a little way ahead still. As is that magical time when you will be forced to choose *either* food *or* heroin and this will be no choice at all. Patience, my friend!

All you need now is to arm yourself with the experience you require and the next stage beckons! You will have, or be able to improvise, much of what you need. Your needle itself may be borrowed or bought from 'your man' or one of his crowd (many welcome new devotees – especially for a price!), or even, if you find yourself in a little crowd of users somewhere, discreetly 'lifted'.

One useful trick if you live in a real inner city area is to take a hammer to the 'used needles' boxes of the exchange programmes and you'll have a whole selection of, as we call them, 'nearly news'[2]. You may even get really lucky and find one of these casually lying in the street. There is, as with all potential difficulties in life, always a way.

[2] Publisher's note: extremely dangerous – don't do it!

Day Four – Hopefully you're all set. If not, you can, as before, repeat the previous day until you have what you need but definitely only once. If you're having real trouble with the needle thing you'll just have to bite the bullet, get drunk, go to your needle exchange or doctors, tell them that you're injecting and that they, by law, have to give you some clean needles. **HAVE TO!** And who says dieting is difficult?!

Because *now*, oh slender one, the back of the beast of fatness has been well and truly broken. Go home and inject yourself with your heroin and that, pretty much, is that. At this stage, even if you don't realise it, you are quite probably already physically addicted. By the time you next leave the house, you certainly will be – and you'll be most definitely aware of it. Because the *only* reason you'll leave the house will be to buy some more. Hence the fact that I call...

Day Five, Day Six and **Day Seven** – The '**Chrysalis Phase**'. You enter this phase, as you enter your house, as a chubby, calorie-guzzling caterpillar and emerge, an amazingly short period of time later, as an intensely focused, drug-addled butterfly positively winging its way to a life of almost-undreamed-of thinness.

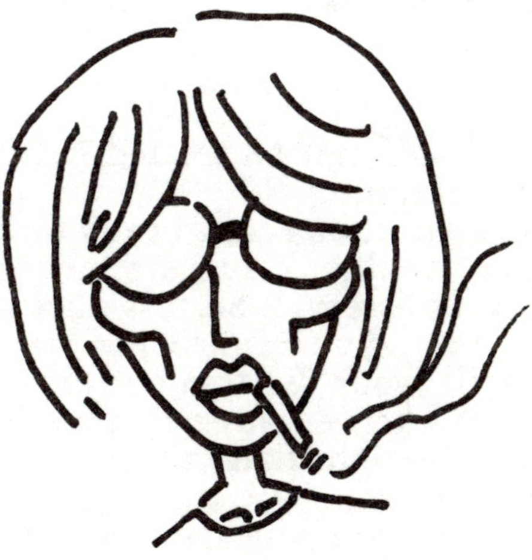

DOING IT FOR LIFE

One way of looking at your life is to look at it in the same way as you look at your body. So, go on, take a good hard look. What do you notice? What stands out head and shoulders above everything else?

That's it!

...It's too fat.

Slimness should not be treated lightly. It's a whole lifestyle choice and needs to be given the respect it deserves. So this plan will deal not just with your fat arse but all the other unnecessary weight that you carry with you through your bloated life: your job (one ticked already!), your home, your family and friends and your possessions.

As you become more focused on the programme it is obvious that possessions are ballast that needs to be jettisoned to maintain the buoyancy provided by the drugs. Consider each (pawn-shop) sale an investment in your slenderness.

Again, this may seem daunting. You may feel that you will miss some of those things, but once more, fear not, for we come back to our old friend, the Diminishing Self-Worth Quotient. For, as your family, your friends and your comforts also start to disappear, your lack of self-worth will make you realise that in actual fact YOU NEVER DESERVED ANY OF THESE THINGS IN THE FIRST PLACE.

Also, by the time you are finally evicted from your house, so that none of those people will even know where to find you anymore, you will be so anaesthetised to pretty much anything that you will barely notice, let alone regret, their passing.

And so, finally, here we are at our holy grail: hand-to-mouth, living-on-the-street heroin dependency. You just DO NOT get fat having made that lifestyle choice. And the best part is that there is simply no going back to your comfortable fatness, even if you wanted to. It's a completely irreversible process and a diet that simply cannot fail.

Some key points at this stage:

- Stress is a major cause of weight loss (please also refer to the Cycle of Anxiety in the next chapter, page 77). Your worry over where you're going to get your next hit, and now, more to the point, where you're going to get the money for it will certainly do your slimming aspirations no harm.

- General hardship is a major cause of weight loss. The cold, malnourishment and sleeping rough are all in no way likely to pile on the pounds.

- Paranoia and general drug-related madness are also valuable burners of calories.

So your only real issue when it comes to maintaining your new lifestyle is funding. And by now you have the biggest asset anyone could have on their side when it comes to raising cash: utter desperation. You will find a way. There is always a way to raise money. Here are some favourites methods gleaned from people who have successfully completed this programme and from whom we shall shortly be hearing:

- Begging
- Prostitution
- Burglary/Theft
- Mugging/Robbery

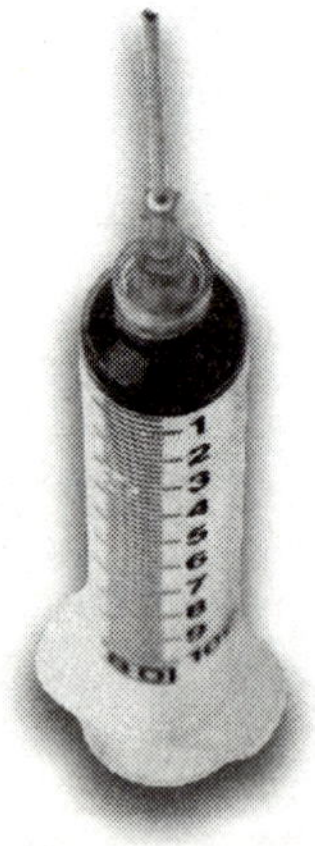

All of these require a little practice, and you will doubtless come up with others of your own, but none of them are beyond any of us now that we've brought our triumphant triumvirate of factors together in glorious co-operation: zero self-worth, total desperation and clinically diagnosable drug dependency.

It is also worth noting at this point that the heroin diet also works to totally nullify your BPF (Boring Prig Factor) – what is more Rock 'n' Roll than heroin?! Whoever wrote a song called 'Stayed Home and Had a Salad'?

Not everybody's journey is the same but we all meet at the bottom of the same slope.

Kimmy's story

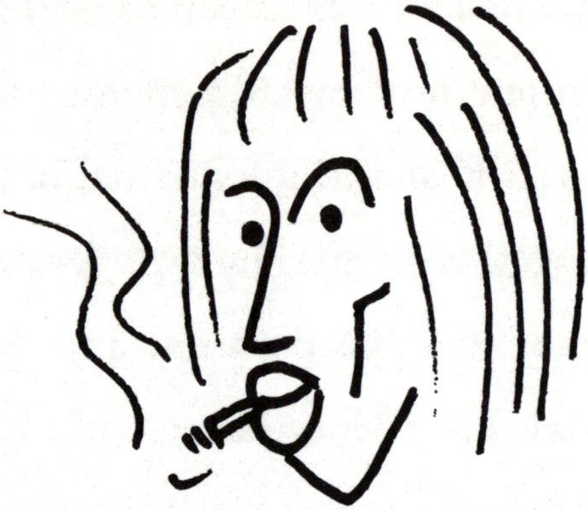

'I was a fat housewife, same as any other. A husband who was always working, a daughter who was always screaming and crying and a fridge that was always bursting. I was depressed about the amount of Prozac I was taking. So I ate. My husband, Brian, never did anything about it. He'd tell me I still looked beautiful and that he loved me. Then when I got really down he'd say that he'd diet with me and that he'd be my support. We'd do it together. Like he needed to diet – the skinny little prick. So I'd eat when he was asleep or at work just to spite him. And I mean really eat. Cake after cake. And he'd still tell me that he loved me. The Arsehole. Eventually I got so angry at his attitude that I started to take it out on him. Snapping and shouting. I denied him sex. He wasn't even allowed to touch me. Eventually he started to get depressed too and tried to snap me out of it, to reason and cajole, to shock and bully. I turned my back on him and my face to the fridge. Eventually he left. The coward.

'I got more depressed and ate more. I began to take it out on my daughter and eventually the courts gave her to Brian. The alimony was cut and I had to move into a hostel as I was too depressed to work. I was 20 stone. It was my lowest point.

'It was the girls in the hostel who got me addicted to heroin. They were prostitutes and drug dealers. I don't think any of them gave, or will ever give, a f*** about me. They're complete bitches but through their efforts and the effects of the drugs, I was soon of a size where at least a few really drunk or poor or desperate men would pay for me to wank them off or to let them come in my mouth without a condom. It wasn't a bundle of laughs but it was a living and it funded my habit.

'After a while I was slim enough that some of them would want to pay to f*** me. Since I was already doing blow jobs without protection I saw no reason not to do full sex the same way. And I'd let them do front door and back door. My earnings rose dramatically. As, therefore, did my heroin intake and the weight has just fallen off. Even those slags at the hostel tell me I should go to a doctor. I weigh six-and-a-half stone.

[Kimmy was not paid for this interview. And won't be...]

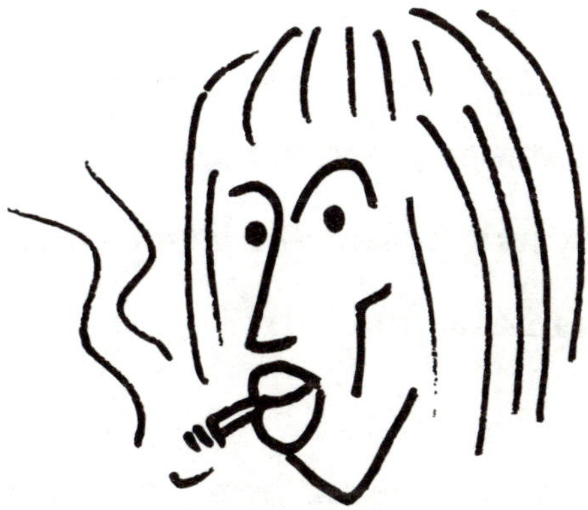

"SMACKHEADS DON'T GET FAT"

Kevin's story

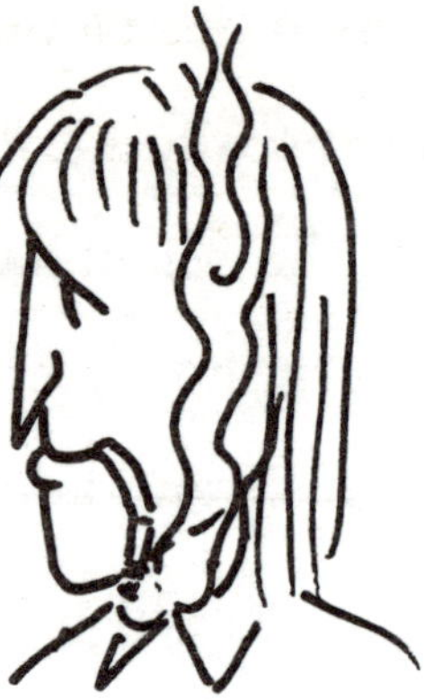

'All me mates did skag at school. I did too. We all did. It was what we did. There was f*** all else to do. We'd rob our Mams' purses, get a load a gear like and go down the old bomb site round the backa Terry's place. It'd be me and Dave, our Barry, Big Barry and Terry.

'Was there that I killed him. Terry, that is. We got into a fight about something, can't remember what. I just remember being really edgy and it was cold I think and he was really pissing me off and I just stuck the knife right in his throat, the c***. Boof, just like that. Never saw it coming. Nor did anyone else. We all just got kinda quiet. Especially Terry.

'The judge said I showed no remorse, but I'd not really been following what was going on like. I was sorta trying to kick the gear a bit but felt that through the trial I deserved a little bit. Was the only thing that made it bearable. I couldn't be considered for parole for at least fifteen years. Life.

'Inside I soon found my place. I f***ed some bloke up in the showers who looked at me funny and gained some respect. The guy who was dealing the brown, Pogo, was a right c*** at that. Very bad advert for very bad gear. So

I started getting me own bought in. Good shit and business boomed. All my lot got right into it. Skinny guys all of 'em and getting skinnier. Me the most.

'One day Pogo forces his way into the bog behind me while one of his bummers watches the door. He was really pissed off about it all. I was really f***ing strung out on the gear. Had been doing loads as business was good and was on me way just to bang up a little to take the edge off like. It'll do that to you. Just gets you a little twitchy.

'I killed Pogo with my bare hands. F***ing nearly tore his face right the f*** off. I was nearly as surprised as he was. And he was really f***ing surprised. For a minute. So was his mate when he saw me clambering over Pogo's bubbling body with lumps of his flesh in my hands. Like I say, you can get a little twitchy.

'This time the judge said life should mean life. Said that drugs had turned me into a menace and a danger to society. I didn't give a f***. I've got my own society and I'm the f***ing King. I'm a one-man drug-machine. I'm hard-wired pent-up glory. And it's the brown, the brown that keeps me sane.

'I weigh nine stone two.'

[Kevin was killed just after he gave this interview... Butchered in a drug-fuelled frenzy. His body was mutilated and hung by the testicles from the second floor landing. There wasn't an ounce of fat on it.]

Jimmy's story

'Ah f*** off you c***. Garan. F*** off out of it. What you got? Whatcha got? F*** off. You got anything? No? F*** off then. Just f*** off you c***. F***ing c***. C***ing f***ing c***.

'**** *** *** **. *** ******* ***** * ******. ***. *** **** ************. *****. ************** *. ****** ***************** * ** ************** * ******

'****** *** *** ***.

'****'

[Jimmy is slim.]

Madame X comments

Smack is such an ugly word, don't you think? I prefer to call it *Dr Miracle*. Thanks to *Dr Miracle* I remain lovely and slim despite my advancing years. *Les amis de Dr Miracle* are always thin!

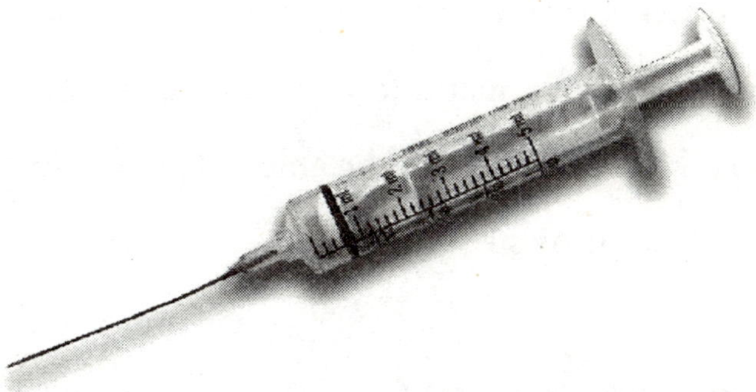

ALTERNATIVES TO SMACK?

It should probably be recognised that smack isn't everyone's cup of tea. There are plenty of other narcotics that can produce desirable effects. The routes will be similar but with certain key differences. We'll be able to go into a few other drugs in this book – mainly where it involves a significantly different lifestyle choice – but unfortunately constraints of time and space mean that we're not able to go into all of them here. Here are a just a few more to give you a taster. I am sure you will be able to think of lots more of your own!

Crackheads don't get fat – When he was still alive Kevin mentioned that many very hardened smackheads in prison, hard men, were ashamed of their crack habit... It'll do the trick and perhaps even faster than smack. Makes you rather wired.

Wired = Weight Loss.

Acid users are unlikely to get fat – Food stuff becomes animate when on acid. *Mr Gherkin is your friend. How can you eat him?* Careful though, don't use dope to get down again. (See next page.)

PCP users (or users of 'Angel Dust') don't get fat – Just way too fucked.

Cokeheads don't get fat[3] – Like crack but not as good.

Ecstasy users don't get fat – Plenty of calorie busting exercise incorporated into this diet!

But, a final word of caution. **Dope smokers do get fat!** This drug encourages snacking and must be avoided at all costs.

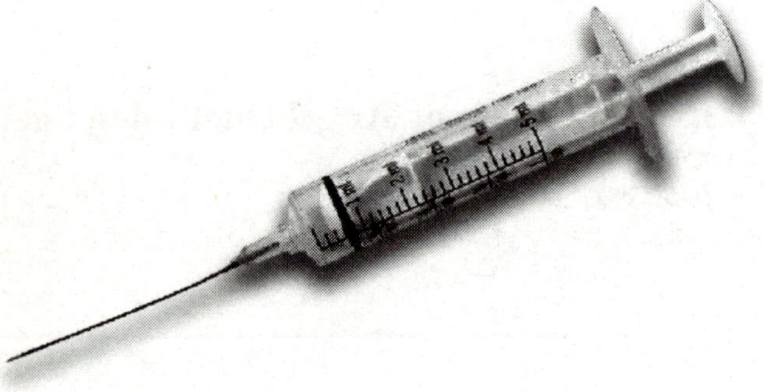

[3] Unless you're Maradonna.

CONCLUSION

So, as you can clearly see, heroin addiction is an attractive lifestyle which is truly open to anyone. It is easily attainable and absolutely guarantees dramatic weight loss. The only wonder and shame is that more people don't have the strength or intelligence to do it.

DIET MIX 'N' MATCH DIET MIX 'N' MATCH DIET MIX 'N' MATCH DIET MI

You can combine this diet with...

Becoming a wino, being a heartbroken man, chain smoking and anorexia.

Avoid...

Narcissism, speed and living in a war-torn territory.

CHAIN SMOKERS DON'T GET FAT

There's been much fascinating research recently asking why French women don't get fat. Indeed my own research with Madame X skirts around this issue continually. Madame, herself, puts her washboard stomach and delicate limbs down to a combination of her busy profession and a predilection for *Dr Miracle*.

Yet, I wonder if the answer might be rather simpler. Yes, she burns the calories through work and, yes, she keeps herself busy in leisure time by her use of recreational drugs but there is something else at work here too.

Why *are* French women so much thinner than their Anglo-Saxon cousins?

Let's scientifically analyse perceived differences between French women and Anglo women.

French women wear scarves and general bits of cloth around their person.

In a controlled test where 100 women in the UK were made to wear French-style neck scarves for a number of weeks their weight remained the same.

French women are haughty.

There is evidence to show that increased levels of haughtiness correlate with reduction in weight.

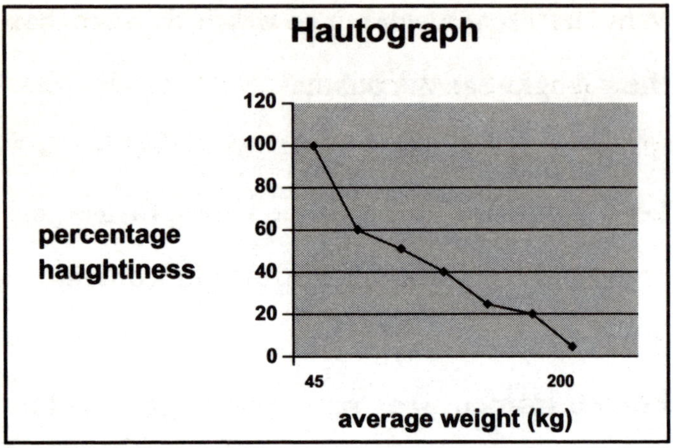

Fig. 2.1

However, beware of drawing premature conclusions. It is my fear that haughtiness might just be part of the **B**oring **P**rig **F**actor found in the 'normal diet' that this book strives so hard to avoid. Could it be that loss in weight causes the haughtiness, rather than the other way around?

Another caveat: How can we be sure that this is a trait of French women rather than stuck-up transatlantic toffs? No, I feel we need to look elsewhere.

French women don't win the right to host the Olympics.

While it is possible that failure to win the 2012 Olympics could lead to appetite-suppressing misery, it is equally possible that it could result in comfort eating. Only time will tell.

French women eat smaller meals and really savour their food.

Really? Do they?

French women only eat the freshest, in-season fruit and vegetables.

Fuck off.

French women smoke like chimneys.

Bingo! A cigarette a day keeps fatness at bay... Actually you probably need rather more.

HOW IT WORKS

The beauty of this diet is its simplicity. Tobacco is a well-known appetite suppressant used by many of the top supermodels, among others.

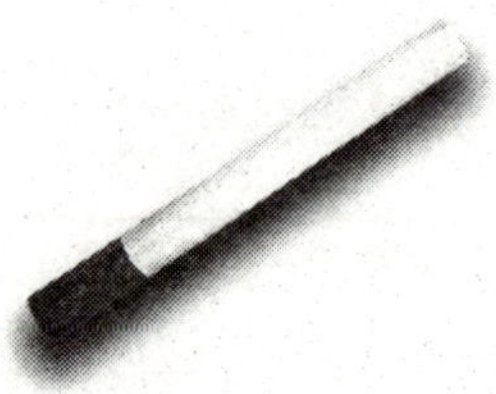

I sense you have a pertinent question?

'But I know plenty of chain smokers and some of them are quite sizeable.'

Sadly this is all too true. Some smokers are using cigarettes in the wrong way as part of a general *joie de vivre*. And as we have seen on page 37, *joie de vivre* leads to a dangerous cycle of fatness.

What you need to do, dear reader, is to make cigarettes work for slimness in forming part of a cycle of anxiety. This chapter could almost be called *Those of a nervous disposition don't get fat*, for have you noticed how very thin nervous, anxious and neurotic people can be?

Perhaps the best way to explain it is to show you what happens when a non-MQQ dietee smells a bacon sandwich.

bacon sandwich receptors + bacon sandwich aroma

= the unholy spectre of appetite

✘

Whereas in the brain of the chain smoker a different reaction is happening...

bacon sandwich receptors + bacon sandwich aroma + TOBACCO

= a WEAKENED unholy spectre of appetite

✔

And so, the chain smoker remains immune to the call of bacon sandwiches and other temptations and the weight stays off! Simple, huh?

Let's take a look at how it works:

THE CYCLE OF ANXIETY

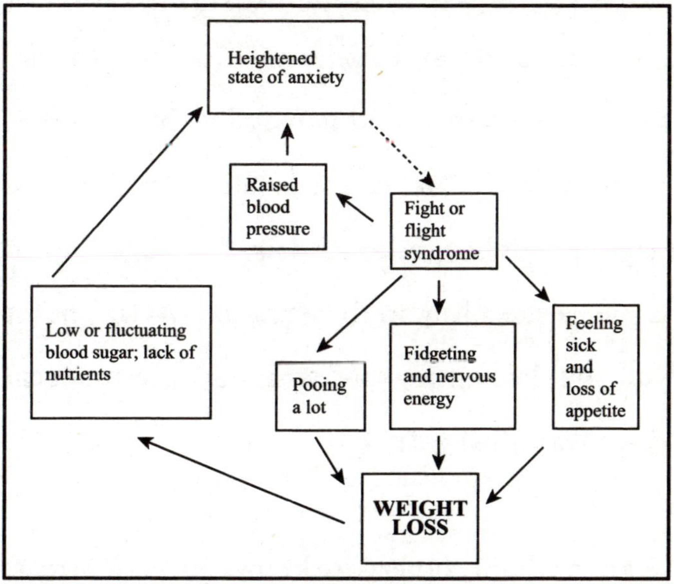

fig. 2.2

'So why do I need to smoke a bunch of cigarettes if I can get slim through stress?'

Why indeed? The answer lies in what *type of stress* you are inducing. Sadly in our modern society – with plenty of food about – we all know about the kind of nagging misery that leads to comfort eating and fatness. This is what I like to call 'bad stress' and is why I've put a dotted arrow between 'Heightened state of anxiety' and 'Fight or flight syndrome' (fig. 2.2, page 77) – it is the weakest link in the equation! At this point you could go either way, and there is a very real risk of comfort eating.

'Fight or flight', otherwise known as 'good stress', is the almost unbearable raised heartbeat, feeling sick, going-to-the-loo-a-lot, sweaty-palmed, panicky state that you experience when you are really really anxious, perhaps before an exam or a driving test.

If you are a person who is lucky enough to be so neurotic that you achieve fight or flight syndrome on a daily basis quite unaided – good for you! (I suspect you don't really need this book and may be reading it only to crow.) Most of us, however, *simply do not have a nervous enough disposition* to bring on the crucial fight or flight syndrome (or good stress) as often as we need it for weight loss. And this is where the cigarettes can help. Not only do they help to suppress the appetite but taken in vast enough quantities they actually work to raise your heartbeat and blood pressure, acting as a catalyst in the 'anxiety' to 'fight or flight' reaction. Indeed we can see in the equation in fig. 2.3 how cigarettes act as a catalyst in the nagging stress to heightened anxiety reaction...

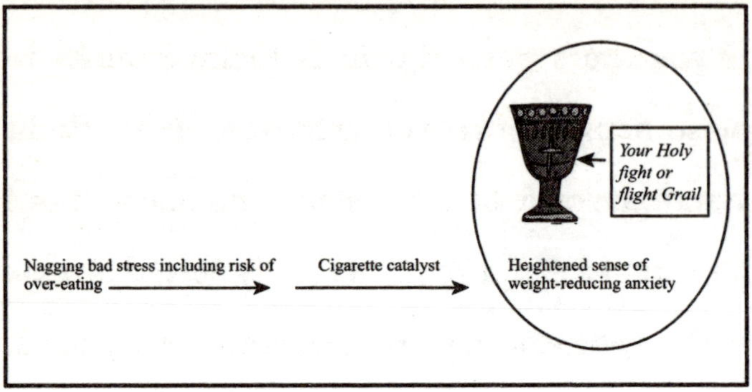

fig. 2.3

As you may have observed from the 'Pooing a lot' box in fig. 2.2, in the cycle of anxiety the initial effects of the fight or flight syndrome can give almost instantaneous and very ego-boosting weight loss – you simply shit out (or if you're even luckier sick up) any sustenance that may be lurking within. Get on the scales immediately before (if you've time) and immediately after a fight or flight attack and you'll see the pounds having literally fallen away! (Who needs colonic irrigation?!)

And, what's more, the miracle cancer sticks can help here too! As well as generally helping to increase levels of anxiety, many a chain smoker has found that there is nothing like a strong cup of coffee and a ciggie in the morning to get your bowels into brisk action!

Admittedly getting your anxiety to the right level for 'fight or flight' can be a difficult trick to attain *even with the cigarettes.* Let's hear from Madame X herself on how to achieve the best results.

Madame X comments

Let *Non Vivre Joie de Vivre* be your motto! My tips on 'ow to make *les cigarettes* work *pour vous.*

Un - You need to smoke *beaucoup beaucoup de cigarettes*. At least 40 *par jour*. Truly you must *fumer en chaîne*.

Deux - Try to find a job that is *très, très stressful*. Become a stockbroker or *tout simplement* find something that you hate doing and are not very good at.

Trois - If you must do sport (and *attention!* sport can dangerously lower your stress levels in the long term) only take up a sport which is highly *dangereux*. If you are afraid of the heights try the climbing of rocks.

Quatre - Whether you be *homme ou femme* become familiar with *la hystérie*. Even if your problem is only very tiny make it into a big big deal. 'ow you say it in English - make a tall hill out of a small mound that blind rodent makes. All this will help you to achieve Dr Harlatan's Cycle of Anxiety!

Okay, so you are saying to me, Madame, I am a very relaxed person. I find it *difficile* to get worried or excited about anything. Well, *chérie*, I say to you that the very thing you are doing - 'ow you say it, smoking in chains - is *très très dangereux*. You could end up getting *le cancer* of the lungs and also attacks of the heart. *Alors*, there is always something about which you may 'ave *inquiétude*.

So when your friends go on and on about 'ow terrible it is that you are smoking so many cigarettes, allow yourself to have the *anxiété*, but it is *très important* that you do not give up, because if you do you will turn into a big whale.

And the advantages of the chain smoking diet don't stop at merely suppressing appetite and inducing fight or flight. Oh no! They are also a replacement snack. *When you fancy a snack you can simply substitute a cigarette.* (It's what all the top models do!) Substitution works on a number of levels:

- Thinking about getting the next cigarette doesn't leave so much time for thinking about snacks.

- It's difficult (although admittedly not impossible) to snack with a fag on.

- If you fancied a snack before the ciggie you probably won't want to bother after you've had it. You'd rather just have another fag.

But BEWARE! If you give up on the diet all of these points will work in reverse! So you really must try to make cigarette smoking a diet for life. That won't be hard though. Although the effects of addiction are less immediately obvious than those connected with say smack, they are, nevertheless, strong and insidious. Believe me, you'll find it easier to stay on the diet than to get off it, so don't let any so-called 'friends' talk you into 'giving up'. What you're really giving up is your only chance to be thin.

To help you to stick with this diet try to remember these invaluable points:

Chain smokers always skip breakfast and have a cigarette instead.

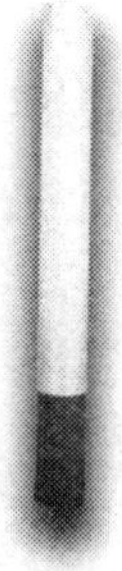

Chain smokers have a cigarette instead of food at snack time.

Chain smokers consume less calories in alcohol when out drinking due to having their hands full.

Chain smokers may get lung cancer.

Chain smokers seriously risk their health and the health of those about them.

Chain smokers get out in the health-giving open air more due to not being tolerated inside.

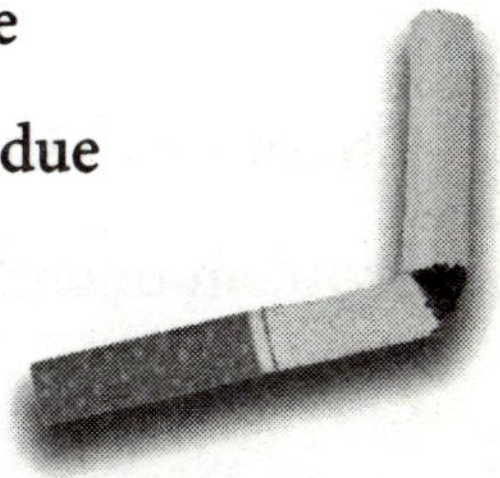

Chain smokers are not always thinking about their dinner. They are thinking about having a cigarette instead.

The worry associated with **chain smoking** helps you to stay slim.

Chain smokers have their own charming community of fellow outcasts.

Chain smoking while pregnant may seriously damage the health of your unborn child.

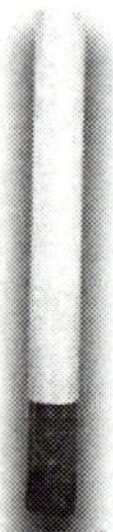

Chain smoking while pregnant tackles the problem of childhood obesity.

Chain smoking after sex is very much to be encouraged.

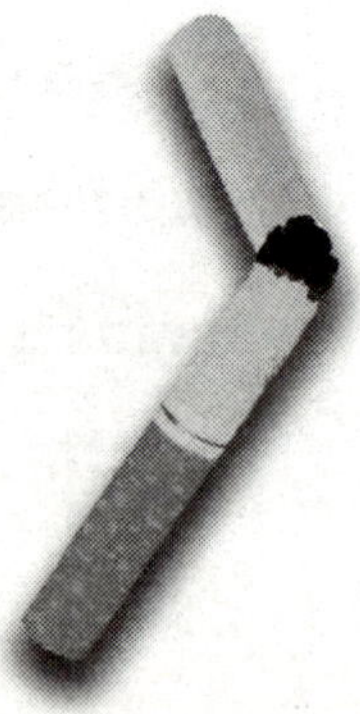

Chain smokers may have a short life but it is full of meaning.

Chain smokers don't bother with 'light' cigarettes. They go for the full tar alternative.

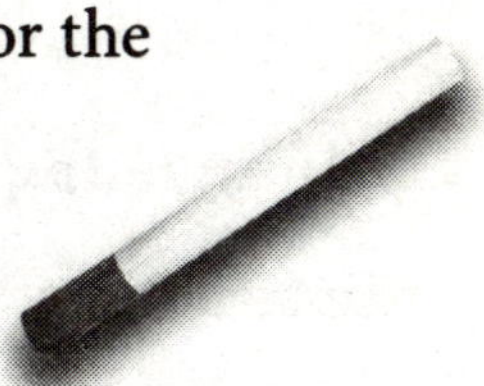

Chain smokers are very handy to have around at a birthday party or whenever a lighter is needed.

Chain smokers are rarely self-righteous.

Snogging a **chain smoker** is okay provided that you have a cigarette too.

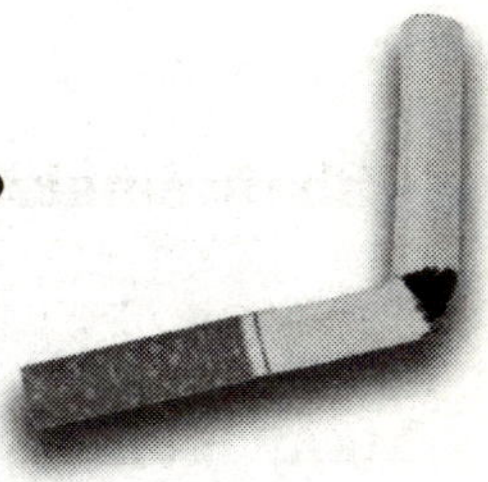

Chain smokers go to the pub more and are more sociable.

Chain smokers seriously increase their risk of heart disease.

Chain smokers don't often get old.

Chain smoking goes well with drinking, drug taking and anorexia.

Chain smoking in Ireland, Scotland and the United States isn't much fun.

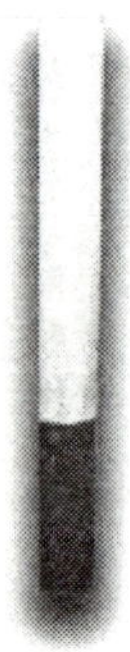

Chain smoking in France is fun.

Chain smoking equipment is cheap in France.

Chain smokers don't get fat.

Many French women are **chain smokers**.

DIET MIX 'N' MATCH DIET MIX 'N' MATCH DIET MIX 'N' MATCH DIET MI

You can combine this diet with...

Anorexia, smack and speed.

Avoid...

Narcissism.

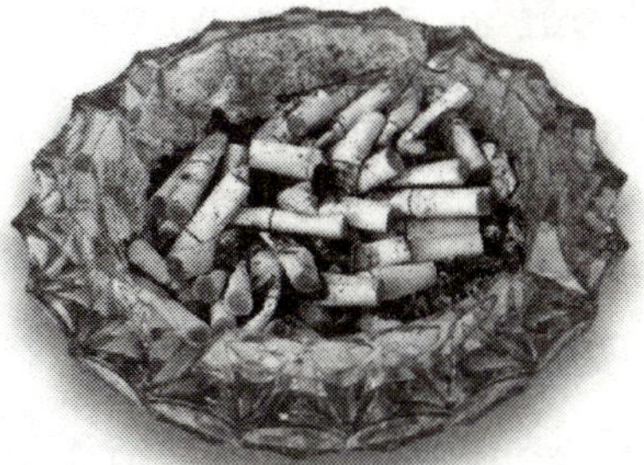

HEARTBROKEN MEN DON'T GET FAT

(A MAN-SIZED GUIDE TO WEIGHT LOSS)

At the risk of sounding sexy this is generally one for the guys. I don't know what it is about you ladies, but as soon as your man has his greasy fingers an inch inside the waistband of his secretary's knickers, you're reaching for the biscuit tin. I don't know why (maybe Madame X can enlighten us), but this is just the way it is. For us men, though, things work differently. The mere thought of some hunky stranger powering away at our beloved's most intimate places makes it virtually impossible to choke down the most tempting morsel. Our stomach tightens to the point where nothing could possibly find a way in. Food turns to putty in our mouths as she turns to putty in his hands. It is an absolute surefire cert:

heartbreak = weight loss.

Sadly this is a diet that is not readily available to all. You can't fake heartbreak. If we could, we'd all be rich. You can, though, significantly increase your chances.

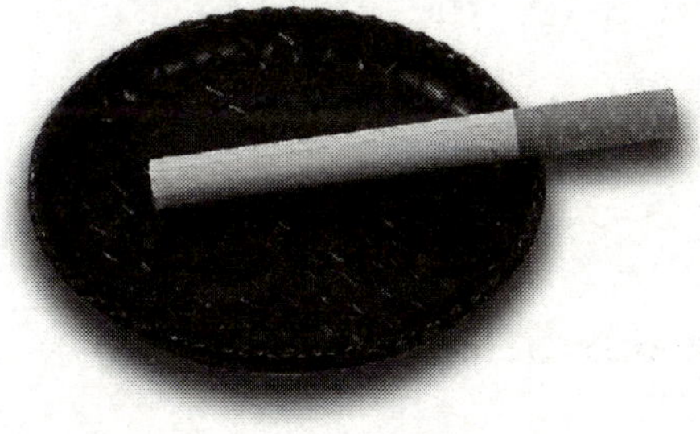

Madame X comments

I don't know, *mes chéries*, why it is that the lady with the broken heart will swell to the size of a big pig while the man will shrink to a little tiny stick of rhubarb. I speak only for the ladies when I say that you must find yourself a lover who would never, and could never, betray you.

Pour moi, my one and only true love *Dr Miracle*, will, I know, always be there for me. I love him so. But for you men, ah, *je ne sais pas*, but *vivre la différence!*

The first question, then, gentlemen, that you must ask yourselves is 'Am I in love?' If the answer is 'yes', then bingo! You have potentially found a portal to a parallel universe where all is the same – only you're a whole lot thinner and obviously no longer in love. (An extremely small price to pay for such stunning results!)

'*But Ah,*' I hear you say, '*my beloved, she loves me so, she would never leave me, never betray me, never find her way into the arms of another.*'

This is clearly utter nonsense and I know you don't believe a word of it. As you and I both know, women are, by their very nature, duplicitous and sexually incontinent. You may well find that simply returning home early from work will do the trick. You'll probably be greeted by the sight of your best friend giving your wife a good seeing to in your marital bed, or possibly your work colleague (probably the one you have never liked and will now have to endure smirking at you every day at the office).

If not your best friend or a colleague, you'll probably discover that the chap you've got decorating your lovely marital home, to turn it into a beautiful nest for your beautiful family, yes the one you've done twenty hours of overtime a week for the last four months in order to pay, is, in fact, taking thirty pounds an hour of your hard-earned money to decorate the inside of your wife.

Madame X comments

Dr Harlatan, have you been at my crack stash again?

The female tendency to stray or play away is clearly shown in the studies of Professor Log of the University of South East London and illustrated in his famous Slagograph thus:

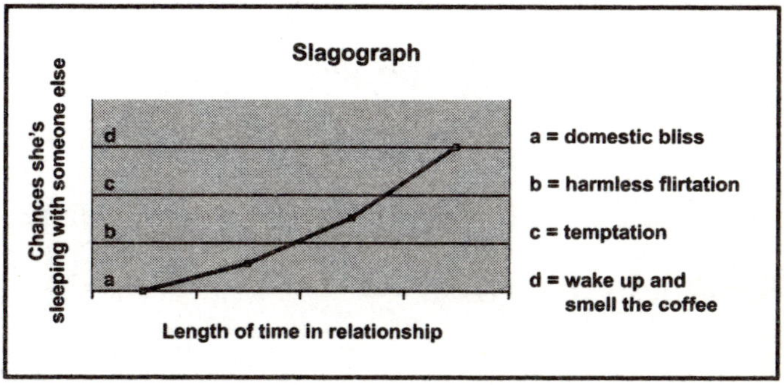

fig. 3.1

And that, my friend, is that. The sickening nausea that will arise as you imagine her screaming his name, of him doing things to her that you've never had the courage to ask her about, of his far better developed equipment, etc. etc. will ensure that eating is just about the last thing you'll want to do. Smashing your head into a wall, sickening violence, jumping in front of a train: yes. Roast beef, Yorkshire puddings, potatoes, sprouts, parsnips and all the trimmings: no.

But '*Ah,*' I hear you say again, '*not my lady, not my darling, not my sugar pie.*'

Okay, okay, let's assume this preposterous hypothesis to be true.

DON'T BE SO DEFEATIST!

Love can't be forced and can rarely be faked. Heartbreak, as we've said, cannot be faked but it **CAN** be forced. So, your beloved would never break your heart? Be a bit more proactive then. With the right attitude amazing results can be achieved.

Try this:

Sleep with her sister. Get the idea? Do it somewhere you're bound to be caught. The marital bed, again, is always a winner. Keep doing it. Eventually she *will* leave and you will be left devastated thinking, 'How did I screw my perfect life up so badly?' You'll be cruising the highway to thinness in overdrive.

If she doesn't have a sister... I've found over the years that almost anybody, male or female, will do. In fact, in tests, another male was found to produce spectacular results.

'But I don't want to cheat on my darling. I love her, she is my one true love, she is my world...'

Grow up! Who said dieting was easy? Just do it! If you *wanted* to do it then it wouldn't break your heart, would it?

'But her sister doesn't fancy me. In fact no one does. Only her – that's why I love her and need her so much.'

Hello! *Hookers* ring a bell? Easy to arrange – just start a penny jar.

> *'But my girlfriend is so sweet. She's so forgiving. Even if I was unfaithful, she'd stay with me; she's a real angel.'*

Trust me, it's not likely.

Steve's story

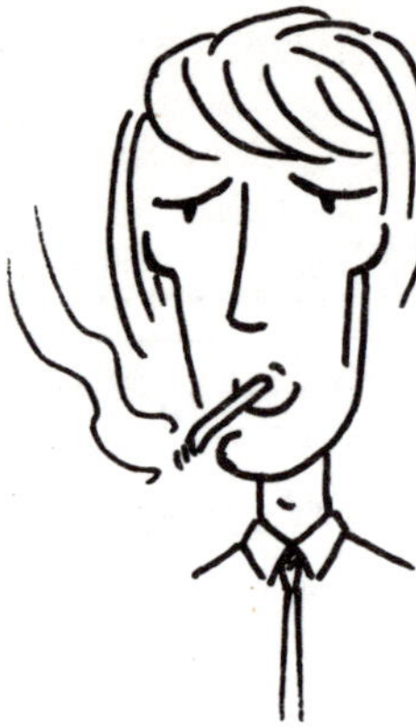

'Life was good. I wasn't fat – I was 13 stone and happily married. Rachael, my wife, wasn't fat either, she was nice and curvy. Womanly. I made good money. We both worked hard. So we'd get home and change and most nights we'd go out for something to eat – a nice meal, a nice bottle of wine. We weren't gorging but, hey, we weren't as young as we used to be and, of course, weren't as slim as we used to be.

'One day I found a packet of cigarettes in Rachael's handbag. Neither of us smoked so I asked her about it. She said she had decided to become a little more 'French'. Seemed strange but I couldn't see the harm in it. How wrong you can be. She started flouncing around being pretentious and snooty. She got a dog the size of a medium-sized piece of fruit. She would only eat medium-sized pieces of fruit. And drink only one glass of wine. I have no idea where she got all these twisted ideas from.

'And she lost weight. Quite a lot of weight. She looked good. Well she looked good with her new French designer clothes on. Or in her Lycra gym wear. With them off, she looked older and had no tits but I didn't say anything. I missed the good times we used to share (as well as the tits) but she seemed happier, well more confident, so I let it go. Especially as she didn't seem to mind the fact that I still had a bit of a gut – she used to pat it and tell me that she liked it. She said I was cuddly.

'The guy she was in bed with the day I came home early (her personal trainer as it turned out, though I had no idea she was planning on entering the Olympics) didn't have a gut. What he did have was his cock embedded fully up my wife's anus. Maybe it was part of some weight loss programme: he was performing an enema on her while simultaneously helping her burn off a few calories. Maybe he was taking his job very seriously. I doubt it though. Looked more like he was giving my old lady a right good poling to me.

'She said it made more sense for me to be the one that moved out. After all, Roger's (it would be, wouldn't it?) place was a little small and I could always stay at my sister's for a while. And it would be such a better start for Roger and her if she felt comfortable in her environment. It wasn't easy for her either she assured me.

'Now it was my turn to take up smoking. It was something to focus on now that I couldn't eat. I was full enough. I had a knot of pain and darkness and despair lodged solidly in my stomach that left no room for food.

'And so here I am, three months later. I've lost my job and my friends are worried sick about me. My sister is beside herself. I wish I could do something for them. I do manage to stuff a piece of bread down me occasionally but mainly I just live on protein shakes – they're much easier to slide past the knot that simply won't unravel itself. I just sit and watch the colour draining out of my life. I just sit and watch the weight falling off me. I'm the slimmest I have ever been. In fact, I am probably very close to hospitalisation.'

See how such small sacrifices can produce such spectacular success!

But what happens if you really are going out with a saint-about-to-be-canonised? Well, if that's the case, there's nothing wrong with helping the martyrdom on a little. I'm not saying you necessarily have to resort to physical violence. All I'm saying is why do you have to be so nice all the time? Believe me, once you start being the real toad that you know you are, she'll start making plans.

Be a real arsehole and she might even get an injunction out against you. Nothing more humiliating, frustrating and ultimately heartbreaking than being *forbidden by law* to see the woman you love.

Madame X's tips pour les hommes on how to piss off your lady friend

1. Do not do anything to undermine her confidence while pissing her off – that will just make her cling like, how you say, faeces on bed linen. I'm afraid none of those comments that you 'ave always

wanted to make – 'Yes, indeed, your *derrière* looks *très grande dans ces pantalons*' or 'Is it just me or are you looking very very old?' will work. In fact they'll have the *opposite effet.*

2. Instead of concentrating on her look insult her *intelligence* and emotional capacity. Something like, 'And I thought *les femmes* were supposed to have *l'intelligence emotionelle...*' will do. She won't believe you. She'll just think you are one of those arrogant mastubators. This is the first step to being shown *où est la porte.*

3. Don't worry so much about your personal *hygiène*. Given that you're working hard at getting thin you'll have to work equally hard at being unattractive. Try the simple things first. 'Forgetting' to brush the teeth and to take the shower *sont très effective*.

4. Being nasty to her pet *animaux* is a *très très* good way to outrage *votre femme*. One little kick at Fido or Tiggles will go straight to the *coeur* of your relationship. (*Oui, elle aime le chat plus que vous*. You will just 'ave to get used to it, chéri.)

Follow Madame's advice and your love will be out the door quicker than you can say, 'At least now I can fit into my speedos!' See how easy it is to ruin your life and break your heart merely by behaving in a disgusting and morally reprehensible fashion? And all in a surprisingly short space of time!

And as you sit in the ruins of your life, full of heartbreak and self-loathing, and with no one to cook for you or care whether you are eating properly or not, the weight will simply keep falling off.

WARNING: Should you get hungry you must stay away at all costs from fish and chip shops, kebab vans, McDonald's, Burger King and the like, and also from meals you just pop in the microwave. Just think of the meals you used to get and pine for them and your departed lady love. (Do not let your mother come and cook for you either!)

Madame X's tips for the ladies or

Les adulteresses ne grossissent pas

Alors, we've already seen that, sadly, heartbroken ladies - even *les femmes françaises et les femmes japonaises* - sometimes get fat.

Malheureusement we are just not built the same way as *les hommes*. So, you say to yourself, "ow I am going to use love and heartbreak to get thin? Love is just a fat curse.' I say *non*. Let me let you into a little *secret*... something that has been known and discreetly passed down from generation to generation in *ma famille: l'adultère*.

I know what you are saying. You are saying, 'But Madame X, we 'ave the boyfriends and the girlfriends too, we 'ave the wives and the husbands. Don't tell us about 'aving the sex. We 'ave it too, so how is that going to help us lose the weight?'

Mon Dieu, since when has 'aving the sex with your husband been morally questionable? Remember, without the MQQ quotient you will certainly fail in your quest.

Eh bien, so you turn up your nose. You don't want to sink down to the bottom. 'Madame X,' you say, 'it's really not *le cricket*. Cannot I just do it with my partner? Could not I just have a boyfriend or do a series of one-night-stands so that no one gets hurt?'

You see, if you just 'ave sex with the husband or the wife you are missing out on a whole world of enjoyable and health-giving exercise. And if you don't have a partner the trouble is even greater...

And *encore une fois* I know what you ladies are saying. 'But Madame X, Dr Harlatan has just told us that adultery leads to the broken heart and the broken heart leads to the fatness in women! Surely you are not encouraging us to go down the passage of the whale?'

Non, non, non! Do not expect a male chauvinistic pork to be always the right one. It is perfectly heath-giving and non-breaking of the heart to have an *affaire* if you keep to the simple rules. Ladies, keep a *liaison discrète* and always aim to have at least *deux* or *trois* on the go at any one time.

We 'ave already seen how *l'adultère* can be used as tool for the men to reach the breaking of the heart. That is all very well, but did you know that the men and the women can use *l'adultère* in *itself* as a slimmer's 'elp?

Here's *pourquoi*:

Quantité – On the balance of probabilities you are bound to get more of the sex if you have more of the people to have the sex with.

Qualité - The sex will likely be newer, fresher and more *vigoureux* - therefore more health-giving.

Énergie nerveuse - Whether it be through the excitement or the guilt you are likely to induce the positive feedback that we see in the **Chain Smokers Don't Get Fat Cycle-of-Anxiety**.

Fumer les cigarettes - *Plus des actes sexuals, plus les cigarettes.* And, as we know, the chain smokers don't get fat.

Maladie - You increase your chance of catching a richness of the venereal diseases. And disease is the Slimmer's Friend.

Madame X's cultural insight

Alors, it really is quite *charmant* how *les anglais* get so upset about a bit of sex *extra-maritelle*. In *la France* if *un politicien* is found to 'ave a mistress he is very much to be applauded. *En Angleterre* he had better keep it hidden unless he wants to get the sack. *En plus*, there is the wife who hangs around looking all doe-eyed and *misérable*.

Alors, pourquoi pas have your own *liaison, ma chérie? En effet*, it is a *très interessante* question.

Did you know that the whole French culture is much better organised for *l'adultère*? French people even have a special name for the mistress! It's '*cinq-à-sept*' or, in English, 'five-to-seven', because that is the hours in which most people 'ave the *affaires*. Did you know that we French scoff at the English in particular for not even having a novel of *l'adultère* in your, *comment le dire*, pre-twentieth-century canon?

Think about it, *hein*? What do you 'ave? Charles Dickens? All the fallen women are orphan-making machines. One little shag before marriage and poof! Gone.
You cannot even reflect on it.
Et alors, the only interesting ladies in the book are swept under the rug in *horreur*...

Thomas Hardy with that Tess of the d'Urbervilles? Do not make me laugh. 'Oh, I feel so guilty, I 'ad the sex before *marriage*. I am so ashamed. I must kill the man who did this to me. Oh *non!* Now I am going to get hanged!'

Jane Austen? If she were not so dead I would laugh in her prim face. NOTHING OF ANY INTEREST EVER HAPPENS IN HER BOOKS. As soon as the young ladies get married - and no sex beforehand - the story ends. Can you just think how much better *Emma* would have been if after marrying that prig Monsieur Knightley, Emma had had a bit of Frank Churchill on the side *de temps en temps? Alors*, she must have got *très très* fat because her morally questionable quotient went right down.

Now, the *héroïnes françaises* are not a bit like that.

Regard *Madame Bovary!* She had affaires and was not fat. *Toute simplement*, she was too busy. And all the *belles* in Stendhal and Fromentin. Adulteresses all! Ah, even *La Princesse de Clèves* gave the idea *considération serieuse*, *avec beaucoup de* fainting and flapping of the fan! *Oh là là*, indeed[1]. I could go on but there is no need. It's just one more reason, which has nothing to do with the markets of farmers, *pourquoi* the French are best and do not get fat.

[1] For more information on this interesting cultural phenomenon see *Adultery in the Novel*, Tanner, T, John Hopkins University Press 1981.

DIET MIX 'N' MATCH DIET MIX 'N' MATCH DIET MIX 'N' MATCH DIET MI

N.B. MEN ONLY

You can combine this diet with...

Narcissism, anorexia and becoming a wino.

Avoid...

Nothing – anything that drags you down is good.

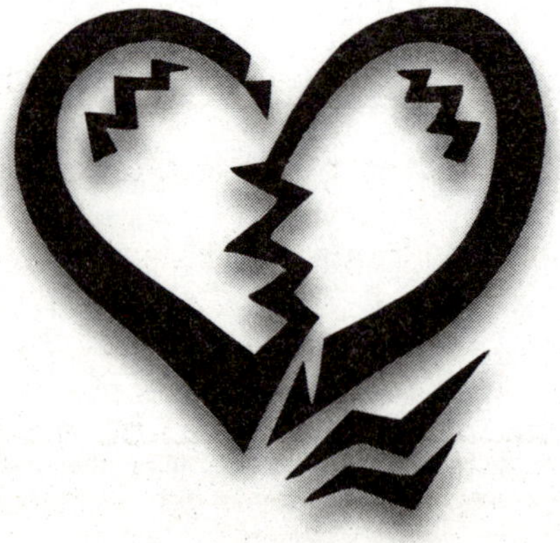

HUNGER STRIKERS DON'T GET FAT

GET SLIM AND GET YOUR OWN (POLITICAL) WAY

Have you tried everything, even violence, to get your point across and no one will listen? In essence, are you just a porker who everyone ignores?

If you've answered 'yes' to any of the above questions the Hunger Strike Diet might be the one for you. The beauty of this diet is that you can get your political agenda across and lose weight *at the same time*. In fact both aspects are really two sides of the same coin and one strand can very much help the other.

GETTING STARTED

- You can get going as soon as you formulate a political agenda that is both not too easily achievable and at the same time worth dying for.

- A good place to start is the controlled environment of prison. The advantage of doing this is that it will be immediately obvious that you are refusing food. If you start on the outside before you've really become someone in the Hunger Striking Hall of Fame you risk no one really noticing what you're doing, or caring. In prison, they have to mind if you starve to death – since you are supposedly in their care.

- Don't fret about the crime thing though. You really don't have to go to prison for very much. We're actually marketing the Hunger Strike regime as the least morally objectionable diet in this book so we don't expect a huge commitment from you in this way – perhaps you could undertake some mild form of civil disobedience[1] and refuse to pay the ensuing fine. It might take a couple of boring months of being given second chances by the Magistrates, Court, but sure enough, they'll bang you in the slammer for a few days if you keep refusing to pay.

[1] Perhaps make trouble at a Labour Party conference or stop paying income tax that funds illegal wars?

- Once installed in your controlled environment the basics are very simple. You simply stop eating and mouth off at everyone within earshot about your oh-so-worthy motives. Just try not to mention the word 'diet' – kind of spoils the illusion.

- **The very best thing to do?** Learn from those who have excelled in this diet plan. Let's have a look at some prominent figures who've had success with hunger strikes, both in terms of weight loss and political impact.

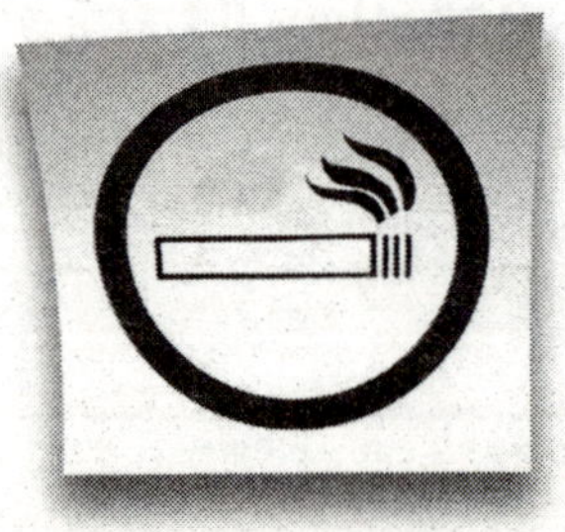

Hunger Striker	**Political Agenda**	**Outcomes**
The Suffragettes	Votes for Women	Achieved votes for women and were forerunners for 'superwaif' look.
Gandhi	Independence for India	Achieved Independence for India and was never fat.
Bobby Sands and others	Irish rule for Ulster	Although didn't get the British government to agree to demands achieved cult status and wide sympathy for political cause.
Prisoners in Guantanamo Bay	Publicising inhumane treatment at Camp X Ray	Full extent remains to be seen but they are generating limited awareness (and presumably losing weight).

THE SUFFRAGETTES

Dieting is quite hard to combine with feminism and normally we wouldn't advise it. That's not to say that it can't be done or, indeed, that all feminists want to look shit. There is, however, a natural unwillingness to look nice to please anyone else, which does nothing to enhance the impetus to dieting. All the more impressive, then, that the Suffragettes managed to combine having lovely silhouettes with important political activity, the benefits of which are appreciated by women throughout the United Kingdom even today.

'Suffragettes' was the nickname given to members of the Women's Social and Political Union set up by Emmeline Pankhurst and daughters in 1903. By this time previous organisations had had little success in furthering the cause for women's votes using uncontroversial means. The WSPU members used 'direct action' – and went to prison for it. In 1909, Marion Dunlop, an imprisoned member of the WSPU, began the first suffragette hunger strike. Fearful of possible bad PR if she were allowed to die, the authorities released her. What action could be more directly effective than that?

It must be acknowledged that when other suffragettes followed her courageous example many were force fed until the 'Cat and Mouse

Act'[2] was passed in Parliament, which allowed for the temporary release and recapture of prisoners embarking on the hunger-striking diet plan. Although interfering with the heroic and slimming potential of the hunger strike, the publicity surrounding both force feeding and the Act had a similar effect in promoting the cause. And of course, the strikers did lose *some* weight, although the yo-yoing must have been annoying for them. For example, it made it very difficult for them to know what size dress to buy.

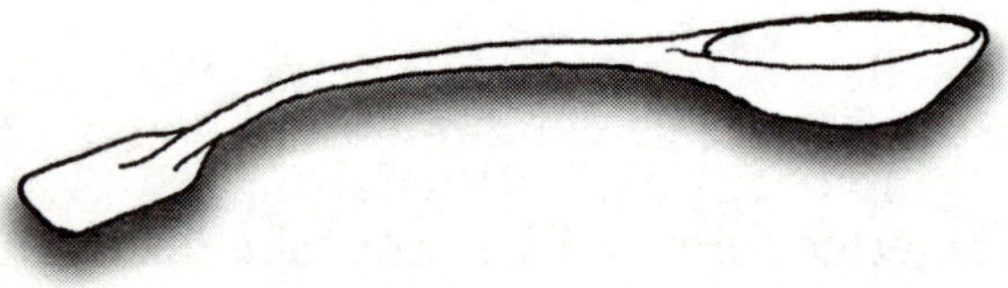

[2] Prisoners, Temporary Discharge for Health Act, 1913

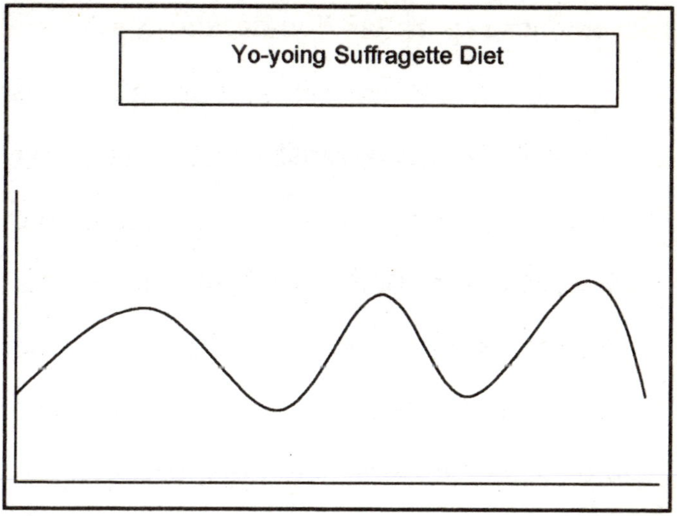

fig. 4.1

Some people put women getting limited suffrage in 1918 down to the effort of women in the First World War and not the direct action. We say to them, how come women in France didn't get the vote until 1944? Is it that French Women Just Don't Help Much With War Efforts, or is it to do with the fact that they had no early-twentieth-century-hunger-striking-women's-suffrage movement to speak of? You decide.

Madame X comments

Non, it is certainly not that *les femmes* in France could not be bothered to 'elp much during the war! *Au contraire*, we pissed on *les petites anglaises* as far as hard work was concerned. We are a *très important* part of the whole effort from *le running away*, right though *le surrender* all the way through to *la collaboration* (the shagging of the enemy).

GANDHI

Truly the king of hunger strikers. You only had to look at him funny for him to start one. And the British were scared shitless of him. (Though it has to be said that they weren't as shitless as the man himself who also swore by daily enemas – another valuable aid to slimming. Get that stuff out of there as quickly as possible before you absorb any more of it.)

The advantage Gandhi had over many was his absolute iconic status and the fragility of the suppression he was protesting against. The British knew that if Indian collaboration was withdrawn, then it was game over for them and goodbye to the beautiful jewel in their nasty little crown. And the most sure-fire way of ensuring this withdrawal of 'good will' was to be held responsible for the death of the Mahatma. They therefore consistently bottled it. Gandhi got his way and remained thin as a rake. Birds and stones indeed.

His only problem was, and here may be a lesson for all of you contemplating a Political-Hunger-Strike-related diet plan, that he was maybe too good. If you finally get your enemy to back off completely, you'll have to find something else to starve yourself over. And just because you got your target right first time doesn't guarantee you'll do it again. Take Gandhi: foolishly he decided to try and stop his country tearing itself apart in an orgy of horrific communal slaughter using the same method. It kind of worked for a while, and he definitely retained his figure, but inevitably someone was going to shoot him, you just knew it. And eventually they did. The surprising thing was that the murderer was a Hindu. The unsurprising thing was that he was chubby[3].

BOBBY SANDS

* Took sixty-six days to starve himself to death in pursuit of Political Prisoner Status. Failed in this, but in doing so achieved Political Hero and Icon status instead. Not bad.

Bobby's problem was that, right or wrong (which is certainly something even a famous doctor like myself is not going to tackle), he did not represent the absolute monstrous overwhelming majority of the population in the way that Gandhi did. That and facing a government who didn't give a damn about him or the Irish generally. He did

[3] Gopal Godse

though, like Gandhi, get extremely thin, have interesting views on the processing of human faeces which we won't go into here but suffice to say his interior decorating business never took off. He did also inspire half a generation of the province's school kids to rhyme 'chicken supper' with the word 'fucker'. Whoever wrote a song about a fat man?

THE PRISONERS OF GUANTANAMO BAY

The main problem with assessing the success of these modern day über-dieters is not just the figure-hiding and deeply unflattering orange boilersuits but the fact that these die-harders almost never get to see the light of day.

These people have all of Bobby's problems only more so. They have even less popular support (in fact their popularity rating anywhere within an eight thousand mile radius is effectively zero) and they are dealing with a government, and indeed a society as a whole, who gives even less of a damn about them. Or indeed, world opinion, human rights, the Geneva Convention or pretty much anything.

They suffer from the problem that they are not only foreign but, more importantly, foreign *looking*, have funny names, a funny language and a funny religion and therefore, as far as the West's government and media are concerned, really aren't proper people at all. Due to this we have little to judge their success upon – they have certainly, so far, largely failed in their attempts to raise awareness of their situation.

The one thing we can be reasonably sure of though is that when someone has to tie you down with a six-point restraint and shove a 4.8 mm second-hand tube up your nose and down into your stomach to force nutrition into you[4], then you surely must be a veritable wee slim slip of a thing.

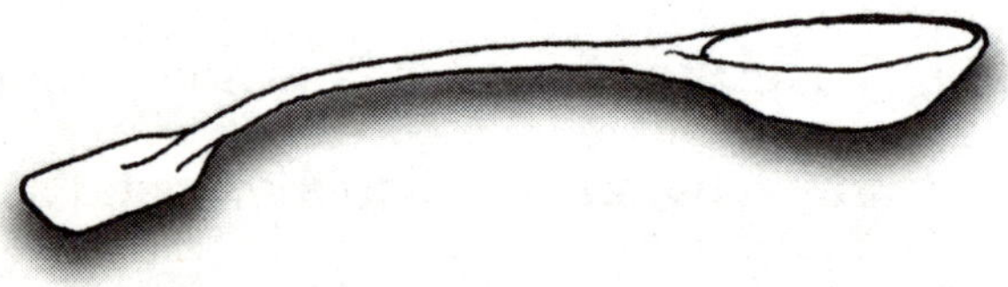

[4] Fair play to the American authorities, though: during the holy time of Ramadam, when Muslims must fast during the day, they don't do this procedure during the hours of daylight. They really are all heart.

CONCLUSION

So, you see, whether you end up dead or whether you end up getting your own political way really makes no odds. You end up thin and that's all that counts!

Finally, you may be wondering how this diet can work since it doesn't seem morally objectionable. All of the famous hunger strikers we've looked at had a valid political point and we would far rather they took this out on themselves, than us! It's a far more humane thing to do, surely? Yes, but come on. Using a hunger strike purely as a way to get thin? That's pretty morally objectionable!

DIET MIX 'N' MATCH DIET MIX 'N' MATCH DIET MIX 'N' MATCH DIET MI

You can combine this diet with...

Narcissism, being a heartbroken man and anorexia.

Avoid...

Smack, gluesniffing and becoming a wino.

SPEED FREAKS DON'T GET FAT

The amphetamine-centred diet is in many ways the Queen of Morally-Questionable-Diet-Land.

STAGE 1

You're fat, you go to the doctor, tell him you're depressed and that diets just don't work for you and what will he do? He'll give you diet pills, that's what.

And what are diet pills?

ALL TOGETHER NOW: **SPEED!**

That's right – the fact that the amphetamine diet is officially sanctioned is possibly the most morally questionable fact in this whole book. You're depressed about your weight, doc gives you speed – WOW!

Yes, contrary to popular belief, diet pills are not designed purely for bored teenagers in seaside towns to down by the handful before they go clubbing. They do actually work. They suppress the appetite and increase pretty much every other bodily function to the point where energy, and therefore fat, is burned up at an alarming rate. You will also find that you've kept your house spotlessly clean and probably redecorated it a couple of times – all that excess energy! The secret is to always exceed the stated dose – this will ensure spectacular results as well as providing two beautifully complimentary side effects: horrendously disrupted sleep patterns and impending mental health problems.

The only downside is that sooner or later your doctor is going to feel that you may be taking advantage of his generosity and may start to ask some awkward questions or even discourage you from taking any more.

Which brings us on to...

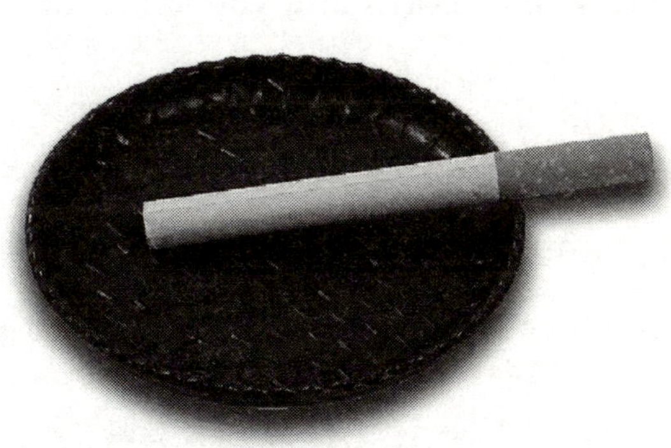

STAGE 2

If diet pills represent the Queen of diets, then snortable speed is undoubtedly the Queen Mother. And the pink stuff is the Queen Mother with her crown on. It is readily available from all the usual outlets (see Chaptitre Un: *Smackheads Don't Get Fat*) and is extremely cheap compared to many of the diets offered here. Simply open up the package that your man gives you, fashion some into a line on your table like they do in the movies (it's not rocket science), roll up a bank note, block one nostril and you're on your way.

You just do NOT see fat speed freaks. It is a medical impossibility. If your first impression is that you've been ripped off and given some scouring powder or rat poison because your nose is on fire and you get a searing pain through the centre of your brain, then, congratulations, you got the good stuff.

Many people content themselves with the weight capping that a touch of speed a day will bring. It really will suppress your appetite; you know you must eat but it feels like such a chore. It will also reduce your sleep down to four or five fitful hours – yes, you'll be out of bed and burning calories a good few hours earlier than usual. But, hey, many people do a lot of things but that doesn't make them right does it? Surely you're better than that? You didn't buy this book just to control your weight, did you? No. What we're interested in is SERIOUS WEIGHT LOSS.

One of the beauties of the amphetamine diet is that at this stage it is perfectly possible to hold on to your job and in many cases to actually become better at it. The extra energy and fastidiousness can be invaluable in many professions – factory work for example.

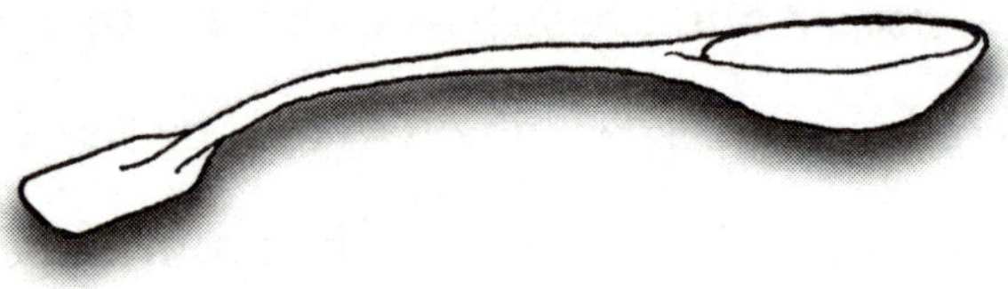

STAGE 3

Here's how we'll start with a three-day stretch...

Start snorting the speed on a **Wednesday**. You need to:

✓do a big fat line before work

✓one at lunch time (although, trust me, this will be a glaring misnomer!)

✓one when you finish work

✓then just keep rolling right through the night.

You can do what you like. Drink. Anything. What you won't do is sleep. A top-up line every couple of hours will do the trick and...

✓a really nice juicy one just before work on **Thursday**.

You'll be a little 'out there' but you'll certainly be able to function. You may in fact be close to functioning *too* well.

Repeat the same process for **Thursday** and **Friday**.

On **Friday** night go nuts. I mean *really* mental. Go clubbing and dancing and drinking and shouting. Start a fight. You have been up for three nights now so increase your dosage and cut loose. You'll find it fairly easy to do; in your rarefied state you'll be pretty damn strung-out anyway. So get out there and burn some energy! For this week you should lay off the speed at about breakfast time on Saturday and increase your drinking. By early afternoon you will pass out.

When you come to, roughly twenty-four hours later, you will probably feel like eating. Go ahead. Be my guest. See if I care. Have a rack of Mars bars, half a pig and a whole camembert washed down with a pint of duck fat. In the grand scheme of things it won't matter in the slightest and, to be honest, you probably won't feel like doing that anyway.

And this next week we're going to start on **Tuesday**!

STAGE 4

Soon, as you can see, you'll progress gradually towards the full-week stretch with all your sleeping and eating concentrated into the back end of your weekend. A couple of months of this and you'll be thin. Really thin. And then it will be time for you to reward yourself for your achievements by truly breaking through to a higher level of consciousness: *Methamphetamine Hydrochloride* or...

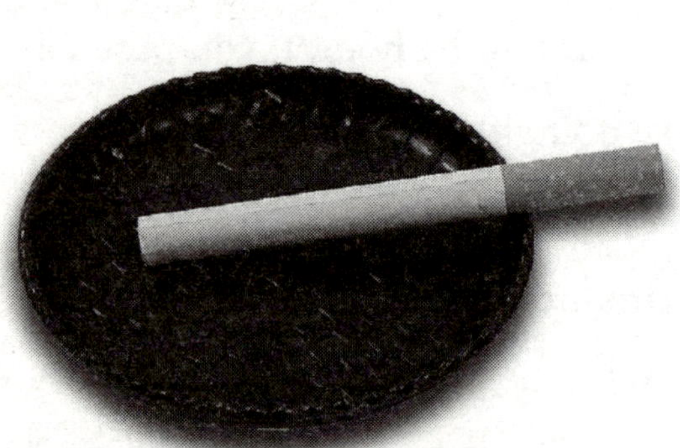

STAGE 5

No more chalk or wizz for you. From here on it it's all Glass and Tina, Ice and Crystal.

If diet pills are the Queen and speed is the Queen Mother, then Crystal Meth can only be one thing: *Darth-Fucking-Vader.* We are truly talking Lord of the Universe stuff here. Your entire central nervous system will be completely overhauled. It will be simultaneously purified and raped. You will be God and the Devil in one glorious streak of triumphant slenderness. You will almost never sleep. You will eat occasionally but it won't even register on your consciousness, let alone your waistline. Your metabolism and respiration levels will go through the roof and, as the weeks fly by, so will your levels of irritability and confusion, anxiety and paranoia. And this is where the pot of gold at the end of the rainbow finally comes into view:

Amphetamine Psychosis!

There really is no better slimming aid, no more glorious a union, than that of the two complementary weight-loss titans that are clinical drug dependency and downright scary howl-at-the-moon utter lunacy represented by amphetamine psychosis. It is, quite simply, paranoid schizophrenia, but thin.

It is impossible to overstate the weight loss potential inherent in madness. The sheer volume of calories that that much deranged energy can burn up knows no bounds. The popular conception though, is that madness is something that nature will simply bless you with at some point or another or not, rather than something that can be induced. *Amphetamine Psychosis* – the ultimate twenty-first century slimming aid – gives the lie to this.

And remember, for those requiring truly swift and dramatic results, the diet pills and speed phases are really not necessary. You can go straight into extreme crystal meth intake from a standing start and, providing that you avoid catastrophic cardiovascular collapse, within a matter of a few short weeks every last ounce of excess weight – and maybe even more – will be ripped from you. You will be like a cornfield after the locusts. You will look twenty years older, have no teeth[1] and be as mad as a snake, but, damn, you'll be thin.

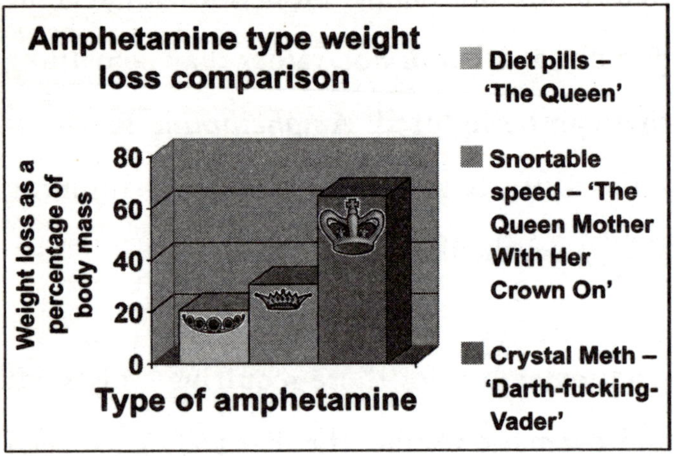

fig.5.1

[1] Having no teeth helps slimming in an obvious way. Smack will also do this to you. If combining smack with prostitution the advantages to trade may be imagined.

DIET MIX 'N' MATCH DIET MIX 'N' MATCH DIET MIX 'N' MATCH DIET MI

You can combine this diet with...

Narcissism, being a heartbroken man and anorexia.

Avoid...

Smack, glue sniffing and becoming a wino.

NARCISSISTS DON'T GET FAT

Ever wondered why very rich and successful New Yorkers or London City workers don't get fat? Why is it that poor people in the West seem to get fat, while the rich are slim? Well, there's one very important factor: narcissism (developing a cult of the self).

Madame X comments

AU DEBUT (Getting Started)

Les Trucs (things to help you get started)

For this *régime* there are a number of *petits trucs indispensables* that you really should buy:

a) ***Les Miroirs*** (the mirrors)

Premièrement, you need *beaucoup, beaucoup de miroirs. (En fait*, you simply cannot call yourself *une narcissique sans les miroirs.*) And please, as many of the ones of full length as you can fit on to your walls. Take some pictures down if you 'ave to, because, *toute simplement*, it is more important to be seeing *MOI* than anything else.

From this moment on you will be spending *beaucoup de temps* making the eyes at *ces miroirs*. It is like the addiction to the small cancer sticks and to *Dr Miracle*. *Alors*, once you start the studying of the self and the obsessing about the appearance, you will very soon be unable to live without your *miroirs*. Your reflection will be the thing most important to you and the looking in mirrors will be *obligatoire*.

b) *Les Produits* (the products)

The mousse for the hair.

The compact for the face.

The small metal items for pulling out the hair.

The face is a good place to start with your obsession. The body will follow. Buy one of those *miroirs* in which you can see your face made *très grand* – a miroir for the shaving[1], *par exemple*.

c) *Les Professionels* (the professionals)

[1] For the full Brobdignagian horror of your imperfection. And then make it right. Daub and cover and colour. Soon you'll look like a blow-up doll. Think Jordan. Think Cher.

The thing that is so *bon* about the diet of narcissism is that, *en réalité*, one needs to focus only a tiny bit upon food. Nor is it necessary to be a regular of the place of pumping iron. *En mon avis*, as a chic *femme française*, the trips to the place for the pumping of iron is for the people with too much of the time on the hands and not enough of the readies. Let me explain this...

Pourquoi pas take the TGV (how you say it, the very high-speed train that is like the Eurostar) while *les autres* walk in a very slow manner[2]. I speak of the suction of the lips, of the stapling of the stomach - *littéralement*, the carving of the pieces of fatty meat from the hips, and the reshapement of the waist. En France we call it *la chirurgie sévère* - the serious surgery. It really is *extrêmement facile*. You are *rondé*, chubby; you take your money to a professionel. He causes you to be asleep and when you wake *vous êtes maigre*, thin! *Eh bien*, now you can love yourself! How do you say it in the world of computers? Game above!

[2] or more accurately, why not cruise past the joggers laughing in an open-topped Mercedes.

It's all about habit...

Has Madame X made it sound easy? I think so, but you may still have reservations. So you've got the mirrors and the products and are cultivating an unhealthy interest in looking like Gwyneth Paltrow or David Beckham (are you Sven?).

But of course you are not quite there yet, are you? You have not quite grasped the love / hate mindset that goes with narcissisism...

Perhaps you are wondering whether to cancel that appointment with the surgeon?

Feelings of inadequacy are very common in the early stages of this diet. Work with them.

Here are a few tips on changing the way you see and think about yourself.

Different strokes for different folks…

The quick change:

For a quick change move into the fast lane. Cast off any friends who are a) more beautiful and b) thinner than you and go hang out with other beautiful people – the sort that really try hard to look that way. Engage a sadistic personal trainer, eat with A-list celebrities and shop only in boutiques selling size 10 and below. And get yourself to a plastic surgeon. (If you can't afford a plastic surgeon, you could apply to *Ten Years Younger*. Or you could marry a Premiership footballer and have done.)

The slow change:

If this is all too fast for you, you can take a slower approach. Start by cutting down on the amount of money you spend on other people and spend more on yourself. The fiver you put in the collection for office birthdays could go towards a glossy magazine. That's the idea. Now, throw out all clothes over a size 12. Also make the important decision to cut down on the amount of time you spend on other people. Why spend minutes helping someone else when you could be focusing on your appearance?

Focus on me, me, me. All the time. I'm important. I matter. Say that to yourself again and again and again. This diet is all about reconditioning.

In general:

Spend time every day studying your imperfections. Keep your compact handy for when you are away from a full-sized mirror or look at yourself in shop windows.

Make sure that the words 'me time, me money, me time, me money' cross your mind at least once a minute. *No I don't care little Sammy that you didn't have any lunch to take to school yesterday. Mummy's more important. Don't you want Mummy to be happy? Me time, me money, me time, me money. You could do with losing a bit of weight anyway, you fat little shit.*

If all this indulgence doesn't work for you...

Don't despair. This self-indulgence will work for you. Go to a hairdresser, a beautician and your regular boutique and make yourself look the very best you can. Then look in the mirror. You'll look in the mirror and think, 'I've had everything done but I'm still not happy. It's because I'm a beached whale.' Yes you're a beached whale but the key thing is you'll start to do something about it, won't you?

Whether you go down the punishing exercise route, the food reduction route (try anorexia), or under the surgeon's knife, it really doesn't matter – as long as you get thin. Only then will you truly love the way you look and love yourself. Don't worry about loving others or them loving you – this will only distract you from your purpose.

'But I feel guilty spending time and money on myself.'

Admittedly this diet *is* expensive but don't you think a little sacrifice now could be well worth the transformation into a new slim you? Come on, give yourself a break, and if you don't have the readies, just get yourself a credit card. Think of it like this. Some people spend their money on fresh organic produce from a farmers' market, eating chicken in champagne and drinking bottled water. Just think of all the money you save by not doing that! Use this handy expression as a maxim: *Less money on vegetables means more money for my nose.*

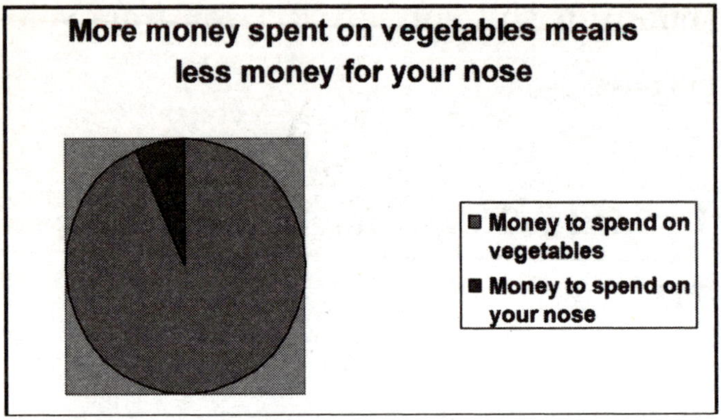
More money spent on vegetables means less money for your nose
Money to spend on vegetables
Money to spend on your nose

Fig. 6.1

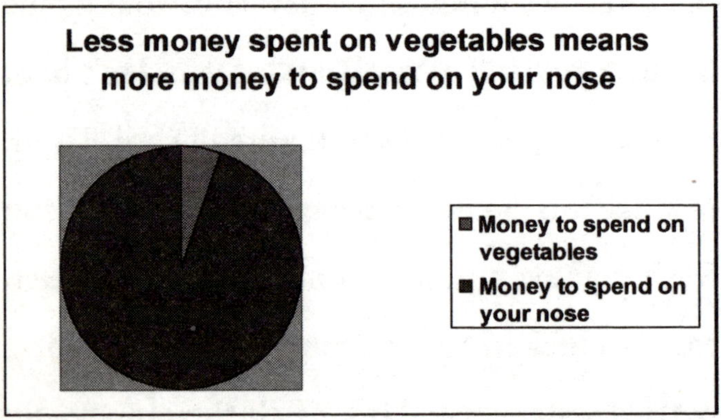
Less money spent on vegetables means more money to spend on your nose
Money to spend on vegetables
Money to spend on your nose

Fig. 6.2

Sandra's story

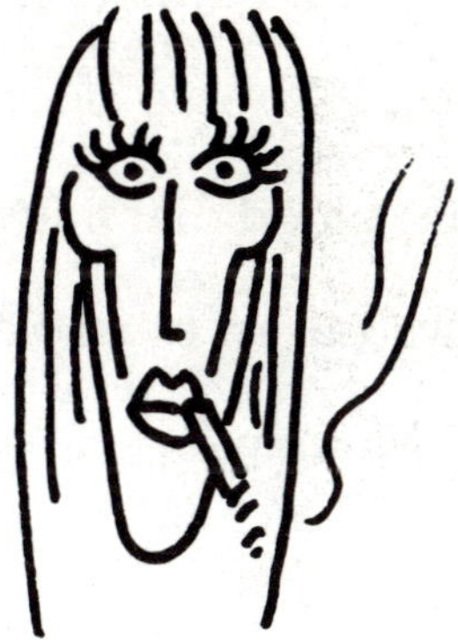

Well, let me tell you about Sandra. I first knew Sandra when she was twenty-five and frankly a bit of porker. A lovely woman but she had no time for herself and this was the problem. It was a miracle that she had come to me at all. That tiny chink of self-regard was all I had to work on. Let me show you how.

The first thing I got her to do was write a diary of a typical day.

She said, 'A diary? I tried to write a food diary before… I gave up. I didn't have time.'

I said, 'No, not a food diary. Just a diary, and you need only give me an example of a typical day. Say a typical Monday.'

'Okay,' she said, and the sad missive below is what she produced.

On Monday I woke up at 7:15 and had a cup of tea. I had a shower, got dressed and generally prepared for work. I just had time to bolt down a bowl of cereal for breakfast. At 8:15 I left for work. On the way to the bus stop I helped a blind person across the road. That slowed me down a bit but the person was very nice so I didn't mind it when I just missed the bus and had to wait for the next one. I eventually got on the bus about 8:35 and by 9 a.m. I was at work. When I get to work I generally go through the post and my e-mails first thing – this day was no different. Then I had a couple of meetings until lunchtime. At lunchtime I had a sandwich and some snacks and scoffed them at my desk. As I was eating, Mike, a colleague, asked me if I might look through a project he is working on. Mike's a really nice chap and it was a pleasure to work with him on something that I've got quite a lot of experience of. At 2 p.m., though, I had to get on with my own work, following up on the morning's meetings. Unfortunately my assistant was off sick and I really needed to copy some articles so I went to the copier myself. Anyway, it's good to be able to know how to do these things. Just my luck! The machine jammed. It took quite a long time to sort out but of course I wouldn't dream of leaving it in a state for the next person. By 6 p.m. I was fairly satisfied that I'd done enough work and left the office. On the way home I remember that I picked up dinner for me and Jim, my husband. I must have arrived home at around 7:15. When I got in I put the dinner on and did a bit of light tidying – the house was a mess after the weekend! We duly ate the dinner I had cooked. Then I put some washing on and paid some bills. A typical boring Monday night really. Before I went to bed at about 11:30 I put the washing out to dry on the clothes airer.

Sadly, it was all too easy to see where Sandra was going wrong. She just had no time for herself. When I mentioned this to her she became very defensive. With a demanding job, a house and a husband to look after she didn't know where she was going to make more time.

I had to work with Sandra very closely to help her see where she was going wrong.

Did you spot the crucial errors?

On the way to the bus stop I helped a blind person across the road.

This is the first mistake. I told Sandra, 'Unless you're Mother Teresa – forget it – YOU'RE WASTING VALUABLE ME TIME! The blind person will be fine – they do it all the time – someone else can help... Someone not as important as you.'

As I was eating, Mike, a colleague, asked me if I might look through a project he is working on. Mike's a really nice chap and it was a pleasure to work with him.

Another ill-judged act of kindness, I'm afraid. The appreciative colleague was not flattering Sandra; he was just bleeding her dry, only she was too ridiculously good-hearted to see it. A golden rule to remember is that unless you get the credit (and the cash) for the work, don't get involved. Sandra should have told Mike that she would have loved to, but that she was just far too busy.

Unfortunately my assistant was off sick and I really needed to copy some articles so I went to the copier myself. Just my luck! The machine jammed. It took quite a long time to sort out but of course I wouldn't dream of leaving it in a state for the next person.

At this point I had to tell Sandra that she really was being a bit of a sad loser and that it was no wonder she was such a fat cow. When she'd stopped sobbing I patiently explained that there is absolutely no need to do your own dirty work if you can get others to do it for you. And certainly no need to clear up your own mess. Again, this is wasting valuable ME time.

On the way home I remember that I picked up dinner for me and Jim, my husband.

By this time Sandra was getting the hang of things. She realised herself that she could have asked Jim to pick up dinner...

When I got in I put the dinner on and did a bit of light tidying – the house was a mess after the weekend! We duly ate the dinner I had cooked. Then I put some washing on and paid some bills. A typical boring Monday night really. Before I went to bed at about 11:30 I put the washing out to dry on the clothes airer.

Again, all tasks that hubby can be nagged to do. I again explained to Sandra that it really is a waste of valuable time doing them yourself. Look at all the minutes that Sandra lost doing pointless selfless tasks! The poor fat thing hardly had a chance to do anything for herself.

Things were about to change. I put Sandra through an intensive regime of narcissistic brainwash. A month later I got Sandra to write another diary for a typical Monday. I was pleasantly surprised by what I read...

***Sandra's New (Narcissistic) Monday*:**

I got up at 7:15 and had a cup of tea. I had a shower, got dressed and got ready for work, ***spending a while doing my hair and make-up****. I just had time to bolt down a bowl of cereal for breakfast and at 8:25 I left for work. Would you believe it I saw the same blind man again but I was running a bit late so had* ***no time to help him cross the road. I'm sure he'll be fine. He was plenty visible there in the middle of the road waving his white stick****. I just made the* *bus by 8:35 and by 9 a.m. I was at work. When I got in, I went through the post and e-mails as usual* ***and did a little early on-line shopping!*** *Then a couple of meetings until lunchtime. At lunchtime I* ***popped to the shops to buy a few essential bits and bobs for self, not forgetting to drop in at the beauty parlour to arrange an appointment for a facial.*** *I grabbed a sandwich and ate it on my way back to the office. When I got back* ***that tosser*** *Mike asks if I might look through the sodding project again 'just because he knows I'm an expert in the field and needs my help.'* ***Cheeky sod, what has he ever done for me? I flatly refused – let him do his own work! Back at my desk I checked my online orders and looked at health spa mini-breaks.*** *At 2:30 p.m. I got on with the drudgery of following up on the meetings I'd had in the morning. The* *idiot assistant was off sick AGAIN today* ***so I left the required copying for the lazy bint to do on her return****. By 5 p.m.* ***I thought I'd done more than enough*** *and left the office for the day.* ***Before going home I instructed Jim, my husband, to pick up dinner. On the way home I dropped in to the beauty parlour to have the facial I'd arranged at lunchtime*** *and arrived home around 7:15. When I got in* ***dinner was ready and Jim was doing a bit of housework while waiting for me – excellent!*** *We ate dinner... I put some washing on and* ***got Jim to pay the outstanding bills. I asked him*** *to put the washing out on the clothes airer and then I went to bed at about 11:30.*

Do you see that Sandra's actually used almost the same template for the day? She got up and went to bed at exactly the same time. Hardly anything has changed! But at the same time she made it into a much better day for herself! But by leaving out all the inessential thoughtful activities, the ones that didn't directly benefit her, she gradually massaged the day into yielding up more ME time. While she was by no means completely at the summit of her mountain – none of the incremental changes so far will help her lose weight – she was certainly climbing the foothills with some determination! From facials and beauty parlour it's not a huge leap to cosmetic surgeon and scalpel and from mini-spa break Sandra will just want more and more pampering – say three weeks in a luxury resort in Dubai and her own personal yoga trainer and ME-time meditation.

Sandra was by this time, of course, a complete bitch. But you do have to make sacrifices in pursuit of your dreams.

But I feel guilty spending time and money on myself.

Strange as it may seem self-hatred needn't be a bar to narcissism either. Narcissism is all about perfecting the exterior to the detriment of inner life. In fact it could be argued that an unbearable chasm of hatred and shame actually fuels a particularly tenacious power-crazed species of narcissism. Never forget that some of the worst narcissistic dictators in history have struggled with intense shame and indignity at some point in their lives. The shame and hatred is merely transmogrified into a handy narcissism. In saying that you hate yourself, you might actually be a perfect candidate for intensely awful narcissism...

NARCISSISTIC DICTATOR (in no particular order)	**WERE THEY/ ARE THEY THIN?**
Adolf Hitler	Yes, pretty slim. Some put this down to vegetarianism. We put this down to narcissism.
Goebbels	Seen by many as Hitler's natural successor. Emaciated.
Saddam Hussein	Before the war Saddam and his body doubles kept a pretty trim figure. His weight has been fluctuating recently...
Pol Pot	A bit on the chubby side but not enormous.

The Ceausecus: Nicolae and Elena	Nicolae was the increasingly corrupt and repressive dictator of Romania from 1965 to 1989. Elena was his high profile wife. Even in later years they were both quite slim.
Mussolini	Again, bordering on chubby but getting on in age of course…
Henry VIII	Exception that proves the rule. A massive bloater. Don't forget that this had to do with his ulcerous leg caused by syphilis. As a young man he was regarded as quite splendid, but cursed with big bones even then.
Henry VII	Henry VII, Henry VIII's dad, was very gaunt. It was from him rather than his mother that Henry VIII got his narcissistic tendencies. But the big bones were on his mother's side.

Charles I	His dictatorial narcissism prompted the English Civil War and revolution. He cut a slim dapper figure. Plus also lost weight in having his head chopped off. There's always a silver lining...
Oliver Cromwell	Following on from Charles I, Cromwell was such a dictatorial narcissist that when he died the monarchy was welcomed back with open arms. Such a killjoy that he banned mince pies at Christmas, thereby creating the prototype for chapter *onze* (War-torn territory diet): *Those living under oppressive regimes* don't get fat. A military man, Cromwell had no excess fat.
Ferdinand and Imelda Marcos	Notorious narcissist, Imelda, and her enormous collection of shoes, played consort to Ferdinand's corrupt and repressive presidency from 1965 to 1986. As a young woman she was renowned for her sleek beauty although it must be admitted that she is a little porky of late. Perhaps she didn't take it far enough?

Kurtz – from Joseph Conrad's *Heart of Darkness* (fictional)	A trader in the Belgium Congo during the colonial era Kurtz was overcome by the darkness of narcissistic dictatorial imperialism. The narrator Marlowe describes Kurtz's last moments: *"Anything approaching the change that came over his features I have never seen before, and hope never to see again. Oh, I wasn't touched. I was fascinated. It was as though a veil had been rent. I saw on that ivory face the expression of sombre pride, of ruthless power, of craven terror--of an intense and hopeless despair. Did he live his life again in every detail of desire, temptation, and surrender during that supreme moment of complete knowledge? He cried in a whisper at some image, at some vision--he cried out twice, a cry that was no more than a breath: 'The horror! The horror!'"* And the unspoken implication is, of course that Kurtz was *very very* thin.

Madame X comments

A good way to induce *le naricissisme*, especially for *les femmes* is to decide to get married. Bridal ladies always care about how they look and nearly always lose weight, whether it be through *narcissisme simple* or 'the cycle of an anxiety'[3]. For the best results - be a bride in serial. Simply marry *un homme* who you don't like and divorce him when you start to become as a pig again. Then get married *encore une fois!*

[3] See page 77

DIET MIX 'N' MATCH DIET MIX 'N' MATCH DIET MIX 'N' MATCH DIET MI

You can combine this diet with...

Smack, crack, speed and prostitution.

Avoid...

Living in a war-torn territory and becoming a wino.

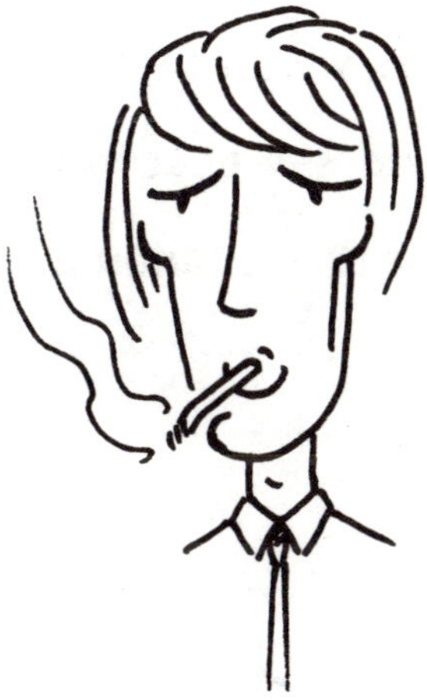

PROSTITUTES DON'T GET FAT

LES PROSTITUÉES NE GROSSISSENT PAS

There was an important work on the sexual act published recently: *Shag Your Self Slim*[1] by Imah Goer. All the means in which you may get thin by shagging are outlined in this book and we need not go into them here. Suffice to say that you are bound to find at least one that is tailored to your needs.

---

[1] *Shag Yourself Slim* by Imah Goer, Crombie Jardine Publishing Limited, 2004

DIET MIX 'N' MATCH DIET MIX 'N' MATCH DIET MIX 'N' MATCH DIET MI

You can combine this diet with...

Crack, speed and chain smoking.

Avoid...

Becoming a wino and narcissism.

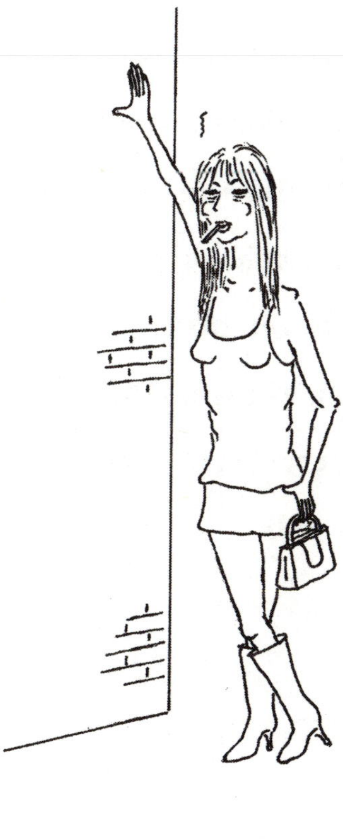

WINOS DON'T GET FAT

Well, have *you* ever seen a fat tramp?

Here's how it works. In general, to use alcoholism as a slimming aid, you need to make sure that any alcoholic calories consumed (and this can be a lot of them) are compensated for by a concentrated alcohol content. Very, very strong concentrations can make you go blind and mad, but this is what the wino lifestyle is all about and should be embraced as an indication that your diet is going well.

Madame X comments

As a diuretic, alcohol is far more powerful than leek soup. Forget spending a whole weekend on the revolting leek-start *régime* favoured by some of my compatriots.

You will find that if you go out after work on a Friday night, get bludgeoned (how you say it, hammered?) and throw up, you will be many kilos lighter on the Saturday. It works every time![1]

You can even have the kebab.

Remember you will probably not be able to eat at all the next day, so have two if you like.

[1] and is commonly known as the 'Hoxton diet' (Hoxton is an area of London where people go out partying a lot).

Given that you will be planning to consume an awful lot of alcohol you will also want to keep the price down. So we recommend that you always stick to the cheapest alternatives available. Going for more expensive drinks also involves an increased risk of actually savouring the alcohol. This will soon lead to dangerous enjoyment of the experience in a civilised way, leading to the very real danger of accompanying meals. You may think that it is only a tiny square of cheese and biscuit with your glass of port but let me warn you now that this kind of cheery drinking bonhomie will only lead you down a fat and bloated alley.

To begin with this diet may seem quite a difficult balancing act, but we think that as long as you stick to the table coming up which outlines drinks to steer clear of, as well as 'Go Right Ahead' bevies, you shouldn't go far wrong. As with the 'Smackheads Don't Get Fat' diet, the hand-to-mouth existence of the true wino will automatically come with time, so long as you put commitment into the drinking side of things.

Superdrinks – Go Right Ahead!
Methylated spirits
Most super-strength ciders – e.g. Diamond White
Super strength drinks – e.g. Tennant's Super, Special Brew
(Absinthe – see page 197)
Anything made illegally (including prison hooch – see page 195)
Ah, Go On Then…
Hard liquor – whisky, gin etc.
Fortified anything

Go-Slow
Normal-strength lagers and ciders
Real Ale
Liqueurs
Port
Wine – particularly if not high in alcohol content
Avoid At All Costs
Low alcohol alternatives -
e.g. Kalibur. Are you nuts?
Champagne
Guinness (because it is good for you)
Any kind of spritzer
Baileys and Advocat (even separately)
Anything costing more than £10[2]
Alcopops[3]

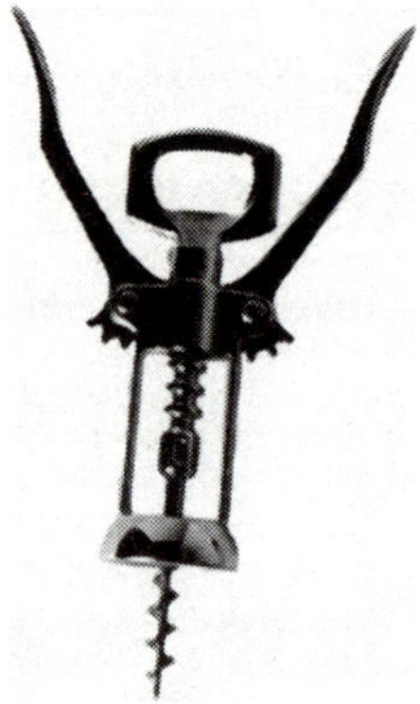

[2] Unless stolen or extremely strong. Preferably both.

[3] Unless underage, in which case acceptable.

Madame X comments

L'Alcool Pour Les Prisonniers[4]

(Prison Hooch)

My friend on the inside, Madame Y, gave me this lovely recipe. The first time I tried it I went blind for two weeks but no matter – I lost *beaucoup de* weight! It is indeed a wonderful formula for making your own haemorrhage-inducing *alcool* at a fraction of the cost of the shop-bought alternative! It is particularly 'andy for those who might have the difficulty in getting 'old of the alcohol, *par exemple, les jeunes*

[4] Publisher's note: Do not do this. It could kill you.

gens (young people) and those who, *comme* Madame Y, are, 'ow do you say in English?, the Guests of Her Majesty. We think you will find these ingredients very easy to get, even if you do not have a big pile of readies. So there really is no excuse for not becoming a *vino*!

Prison Hooch Recipe:

Ingredients:

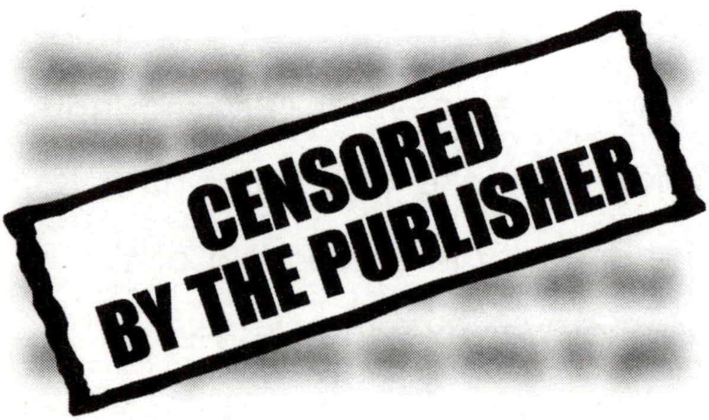

Method:

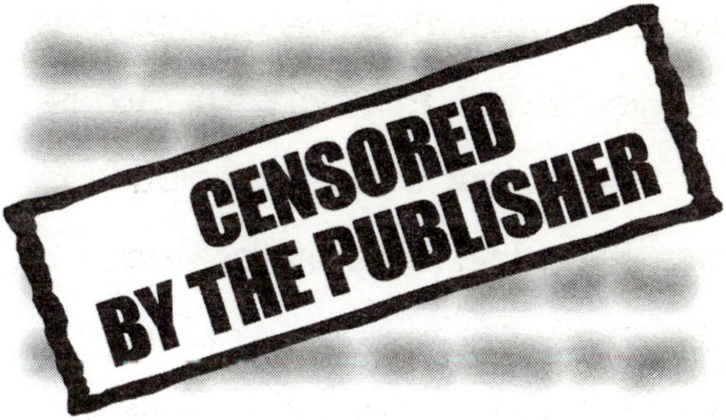

Et voilà! Consume and go blind. What could be *plus simple*?

Madame X comments

If you want to embark on *le régime du vino* go to the home of *le vin*! My homeland is a very good place indeed to embark on your lifestyle choice of *le vino*. Did you know that in the French supermarkets you can buy whole cartons of *le vin rouge* for less than €1? This *vin* is so *terrible* that it aids the dieting by dissolving the lining of *l'estomac*.

And did you know that *la France* is also the home of very strong drinks indeed - none stronger and more of a strain on the eyesight than *la fée verte elle-même: l'absinthe*. The absinthe can be made in the many different ways but the basic rule is that it is made from *l'alcool très très fort* (the very very strong alcohol), which is then made even *plus fort* (more strong). The true *absinthe* has a substance called the wormwood in it, which helps with the hallucinations - an extra help when losing the weight[5]. Even without the wormwood, the strength of this drink all alone will mean that one is *incapable* of finding the dinner.

The use of the absinthe as a slimming aid was *très populaire* among the fashionable *artistes* of the past - many of them 'aving a connection to *la France*. The famous persons taking *l'absinthe* include Verlaine, Rimbaud, Hemmingway, Toulouse-Lautrec and Oscar Wilde. Manet,

[5] See page 67 'Acid users are unlikely to get fat'.

Degas and Picasso drew pictures of their favourite absinthe drinkers[6], who were thin of course, and I'm sure these *artistes* had *un petit peu* themselves! *Mais le plus célèbre* drinker *de tout*? Vincent van Gogh. I urge you to go and look at his interesting paintings. Do you think this was a man concerned with his food? Did this man have a general *joie de vivre* that caused him to get fat? *Le fou? Oui.* Without ear? *Partialement.* Inspired? *Certainement.* 'aving the worry about a large spaghetti bolognese? *Non!*

[6] All of the subjects depicted drinking absinthe are extremely thin. Our favourite is the Picasso 1901 Melville Hall, New York, specimen.

Toute simplement no respectable French *vino* would be without the absinthe.

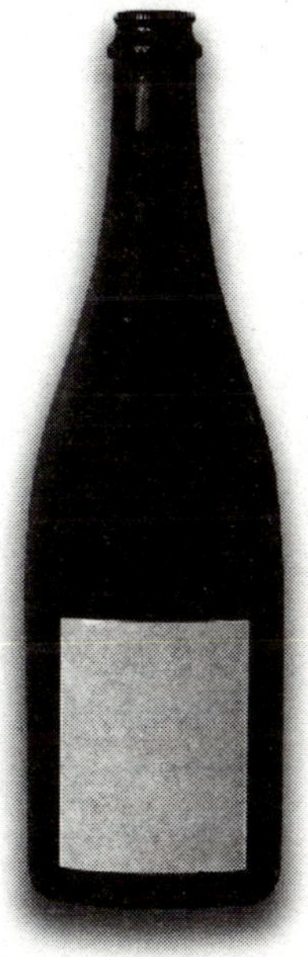

DIET MIX 'N' MATCH DIET MIX 'N' MATCH DIET MIX 'N' MATCH DIET MI

You can combine this diet with...

Crack, chain smoking and glue sniffing.

Avoid...

Narcissism and living in an impoverished and war-torn territory[7].

[7] Especially not with absinthe drinking, as wormwood is known to help get rid of tapeworms.

GLUE SNIFFERS DON'T GET FAT

It's a sad truth that the creeping curse of fatness has now reached the under 16s. You may have noticed as you make your way through the fat-field of the modern world quite how many of today's school children are overweight. Youth obesity is today's scourge of the playground. Where we used to have polio, whooping cough and measles, we now have fatness, overeating and MORE FATNESS.

FACT: 100% of overweight children get bullied. And if they wear glasses you can double that.

You may also have noticed that, almost without exception, traditional diet plans are aimed exclusively at adults. So, if you're an overweight youngster or indeed the parent of a fat child, what do you do? The answer may be simpler than you think.

IF YOU'RE READING THIS BOOK AS A YOUNG PERSON...

Fret-not oh youthful reader, you have not been forgotten. You have not been condemned to an adolescence of bloated porkiness until you can afford some hard drugs. There is an easy, affordable solution: glue.

Although not in itself such a valuable slimming aid as, for example, speed, it is very much a step in the right direction. Don't look at it as a 'poor man's' version of some other diet in this book. Embrace and enjoy your youth (trust us oldies here, it will soon fly by); there'll be plenty of time for heroin or crystal meth when you're older. If you give it a go, you'll find that, maybe contrary to your pre-conceptions, you can get pretty severely mashed up on glue.

It is also extremely easy to get yourself started on the programme. All you need is a plastic bag and some glue and you're all set.

Here's some I prepared earlier!

Just remember to add the glue before you add your face. Breathe long, hard and deep and off you go.

Glue works as a slimming aid in an extremely simple yet effective way: it will render you just way too wasted to even contemplate anything as downright complicated as finding anything to eat, let alone trying to choke it down.

Use something strong.

✓Tile Adhesive

✓Mounting Glue

✓Multi-purpose Bonding Cement

All good. But Gloy Gum = bad.

N.B. Be extremely careful when using Superglue, unless you want to spend the rest of your life with a Tesco carrier bag as a face. Not that that's done too badly for Michael Jackson.

And you will be reptilian! You will veer from pure aggression to dull stupidity. Your face will be taken off, your brain removed and your face jammed forcibly back into place. You may find yourself lying in dog faeces behind a car park. You may find yourself with your hands in your best friend's kid sister's knickers. You will *not* find yourself in the Indian takeaway.

ADVICE FOR MUMS AND DADS...

Naturally you, as caring parents, don't want to suffer the sight of darling Wayne or Jocasta as a little barrel, but what can you do about it? If normal dieting in adults is hard enough because of the lack of will power to follow a morally sound regime, the problem is magnified to the power of ten in youngsters, who, given half the chance, would spend their days eating 'cola bottles' in front of the television.

Well, when helping your little one to lose weight, why not harness some of that devil-may-care, childish bloody-mindedness by getting them to do so the morally questionable way?

Understandably you may baulk at some of the more extreme diets in this book. Heroin addiction and prostitution are probably best left until later in life. What is more, drugs administered to children can actually produce the opposite effects to those experienced by adults. A drug very similar to speed is actually used in children to calm them down and would obviously not produce the required dieting results. There's always alcoholism, but again this is hard for children. They really don't like the taste of the stuff and it's unlikely that they would ever self-administer. Also, access to drink outside the home is tricky for the under 10s. Furthermore, the logistical problems in sending a child to a war-torn territory (see page 228) may be insurmountable.

This is why we've created a Morally Questionable Diet tailored to the needs of younger sufferers. Like many of the diets in this book, the beauty of the regime is in its simplicity. Like smack, once the problem of initial supply is overcome the programme very much takes care of itself. And, of course, your child has the advantage of YOU, their parents, being prepared to buy them their very first fix and to keep them supplied at any points in the future.

Let's see how you can help your child to diet with the following action plan.

ACTION PLAN

Day 1

Buy your child some solvent-based product. It doesn't necessarily have to be glue. The key thing is that it should be one of the solvent-based items marked with warnings.

Encourage the child to sniff the product. Demonstrate how with long, deep, yogic inhalations.

Day 2 (and forever)

Sit back and marvel as your healthy chubby cherub becomes a wraith-like, blank, sullen, dishonest, thieving shadow of their former self.

DOING IT FOR LIFE

Honestly? They probably won't. If the blighters make it to adulthood they'll probably go on to the more regular adult drugs of smack, crack and speed etc.

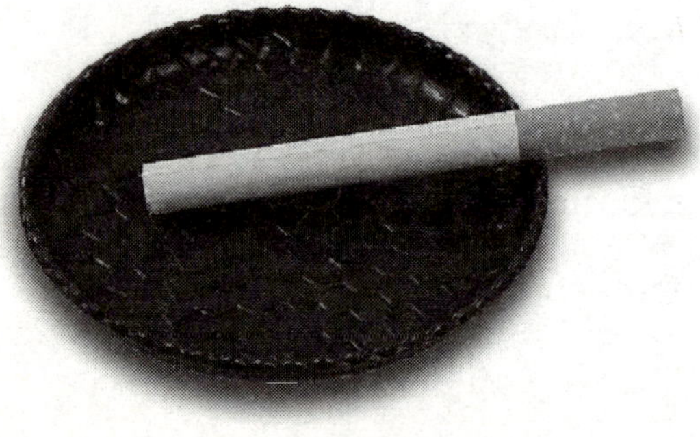

Gavin's story

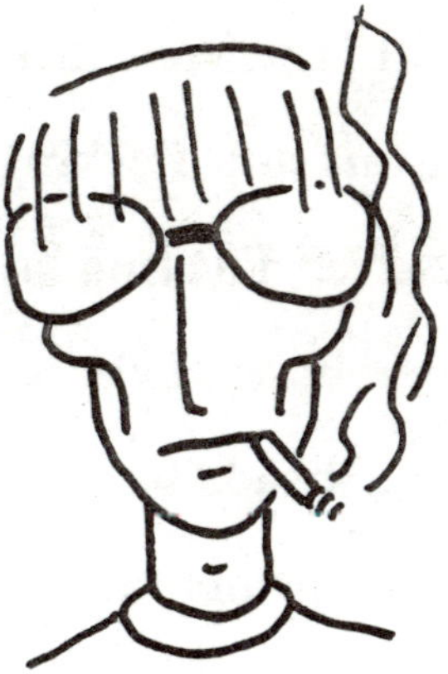

'It's like whoooooa man. Just fucking booooof. First time thought my fucking eyes were bleeding. And this rushing noise. Like dropping through a fucking air tunnel or something. Fucking brilliant. Blinding. Nearly fucking pissed myself. Not laughing. Just nearly pissed myself. One time I did actually shit my pants. We all fucking pissed ourselves. I couldn't fucking stand I was so wacked and laughing so much. I just lay on the concrete and rips my kecks off over the top of my shoes. My jeans weren't that shitty so it was alright. We chucked the pants at this granny at a bus stop. Fucking brilliant man. We pissed ourselves. Fucking brilliant. We just do shit like that all day. Lying around fucking rushing with our heads banging and banging and like yeah so out there it's not fucking true man. We don't eat or nothing just do glue and piss ourselves and fuck about. Pete tried to drive his brother's car one time when we was doing it. Went straight into a fucking wall. Killed himself fucking hell. We just pissed ourselves and legged it. Not laughing.

'And the next day you can't eat or nothing neither. Your mouth hurts like fuck man. Really sore. Like raw. That and sick. Pretty fucking 'gaggy you get. That and the fucking headache. Man.

'Yeah guess we're all pretty thin. Those of us that's left.'

DIET MIX 'N' MATCH DIET MIX 'N' MATCH DIET MIX 'N' MATCH DIET MI

You can combine this diet with...

Chain smoking and becoming a wino.

Avoid...

Narcissism and hunger striking.

ANOREXICS DON'T GET FAT

Do you think that you can't cope with moderation or limitation? Are you fed up with the rules and regulations that other diets, including those in this book, impose? Too many friends? Do you want to simplify life?

Well, why not try slimming the al-Qaida way? The anorexia diet might be just the thing. For truly this is the fundamentalist mother-of-all-diets. There's no faffing around with 'cutting down' or 'cutting back'. It's an all or nothing suicide mission and, done properly, there's no way back! All you need to do is give yourself over to the cause. Before long, you'll be as thin as you like and will have lost most of your friends.

A word of warning though: Once embarked upon, it requires a lifetime of dedication. Verily unto the end. If you go back on it you will almost certainly become fatter than ever before. For this reason anorexia might be a diet to be approached later in life. Also, if you are a teenager or young woman, please be aware that it's really rather clichéd to do anorexia. Cliché has been known to reduce the **M**orally **Q**uestionable **Q**uotient. If something is expected of you, it is not so morally questionable. I prefer to think of the anorexic diet as a super-regime for someone a bit like a fat, gruff, middle-aged politician, known to enjoy consumption, a punch-up and the odd round of croquet. Someone for whom shagging might not be enough on its own.

FAT POLITICIAN'S PARLIAMENTARY YOU ARE NOT WHAT YOU DON'T EAT™ ANOREXIA DIARY

Monday

Fat Politician weighs himself.

Stick of celery.

Fat Politician meets with top civil servant responsible for Transport (ongoing silent regime of 500 bum squeezes).

Other governmental business.

Tuesday

Fat Politician weighs himself before drinking 3 litres of water.

Fat Politician goes on seven-mile run.

Fat Politician signs off on Statutory Implement incorporating EU Directive 7/32 into United Kingdom law.

TREAT! Fat Politician has an apple. (60 calories – allowed because of the run.)

Other business – consultations with personal parliamentary secretary over various constituency problems.

Wednesday

Fat Politician jogs to Prime Minister's Question Time.

Prime Minister's Question Time.

Fat Politician power walks back to office

(a bit too tired now for jogging).
Otherwise similar to Monday
and Tuesday.
Eats nothing.

Thursday

Fat Politician weighs himself. A bit depressed because hasn't lost as much weight as last week.
Fat Politician drops Carol Vordeman's Detox Diet whilst making a controversial speech on ASBOs in the House of Commons.
Fat Politician's suspected eating disorder is discussed on *Newsnight*.

Friday

Diet similar to Monday and Tuesday.
Onion may be substituted for celery.

If time, five-mile jog in the heat of the midday sun. If no time, ongoing regime of silent leg lifts.

TREAT! Vodka and orange. (Very high in calories but glamorous anorexic drink so allowed.)

Saturday

Fat Politician writes *My Battle with Anorexia* article for *Hello!*

Eats nothing.

Sunday

Fat Politician weighs himself.

TREAT! Fat Politician watches *The Karen Carpenter Story* (simultaneous leg lifts).

Sunday lunch is a cucumber lightly smeared with marmite.

HOW IT WORKS

Put simply: you don't eat; you get thin. It's a little bit like the hunger-striking diet except there is no political agenda. Your body becomes the world and your slimness *is* the political agenda. It's a good one for those with little imagination or who are simply bored of their causes and no longer terribly interested in the outside world. No philosophies to espouse, no drugs dealers to navigate, you don't even need to go to the corner shop to buy a packet of ciggies.

Ideally you want to avoid food altogether and do so as conspicuously as possible. However, it is sometimes difficult to prevent all food morsels from passing your lips, especially if you choose to do it without drugs, cigarettes and chewing gum (Anna's Little Helpers).

- Only eat food that takes more calories to consume than it gives you in energy – examples are radishes, celery, cucumber and spring onions. Lettuce is probably okay too if eaten in moderation.

- There is always the option of sicking up. However, don't overuse this facility. Something is bound to get into your system and there is some proof that making yourself sick speeds up the body's absorption rate.

- Go ahead with laxatives!

- New research has shown that if you eat your food in the French language calorie intake is roughly halved (kcal + French = ½).

Madame X comments

Some English to French translations of common anorexic foods.

Celery - *le céleri*

Cucumber - *le concombre*

Radish - *le radis*

Onion - *l' oignon.*

DOING IT FOR LIFE

See pages 218-221.

And don't forget, the anorexia diet, if done properly, will seriously reduce your life expectancy. So no worrying about piling on the pounds as you get older!

BUT IS IT MORALLY QUESTIONABLE?

Anorexia nervosa is a psychological condition and not morally questionable *per se*. To consciously decide to become anorexic in order to lose weight probably *is* morally questionable.

Madame X comments

People think that *l'anorexie* is a *moderne* phenomenon. I am not quite in the agreement. I think if you look back through the ages you may recognise that a number of people got involved with the anorexia plan - mostly bored and frustrated upper class women. Consider Cathy in *Wuthering Heights*. What exactly did she die of? Love? *Pah!* And was she a great fatty? Many young women die in Dickens too. You tell me it's consumption. How did they get consumption? By being too thin! Also, my favourite, Emma Bovary, drank vinegar to get thin - a sure sign of an *anorexique* at work. So, you see, there is a long and venerable *histoire*.

DIET MIX 'N' MATCH DIET MIX 'N' MATCH DIET MIX 'N' MATCH DIET MI

You can combine this diet with...

Chain smoking, smack, speed, narcissism and being a heartbroken man.

Avoid...

Glue sniffing and becoming a wino.

RESIDENTS OF WAR-TORN IMPOVERISHED TERRITORIES DON'T GET FAT

It has, as I'm sure you're aware, been claimed that women of certain countries 'don't get fat'. Although this is obviously quite a bold, and clearly questionable, claim let's assume, for the sake of argument, that it is true. That the women of a couple of the world's most highly-developed and down-right rich nations *don't get fat*. Okay, well how does that help you? Let's face it; it doesn't. So Madame or Japanese-Lady-sama (and whoever else doesn't get fat), you don't get fat? Well bully for you! I'm so happy for you. Nice to see you looking so smug and thin and making a whole load of money by persuading the rest of us that we can suddenly become you. It D-O-E-S-N'-T W-O-R-K. You can no more suddenly become French than you can suddenly become a banana and however much money you hand over in the process of denying this fact, it remains just that: a fact. For those of us born and raised as pie-eating lovers-of-life, nothing is suddenly going to turn us into the opposite: repressed and withered old shrews who order a big old hunk of cake and then surreptitiously return it uneaten to the waiter. I mean, purrlease!

And it's not even as if a bit of relocation is going to help. Were we to turn up, suitcase in hand, in downtown Paris or Tokyo, we wouldn't suddenly become a different person. They still have FOOD in these places for God's sake! You can still wake up hungry in the night and go out and get a few Big Macs rammed down your porky little face.

And the time, effort and money required to *pretend* to be one of these people… really! Let's look at how that works in practice.

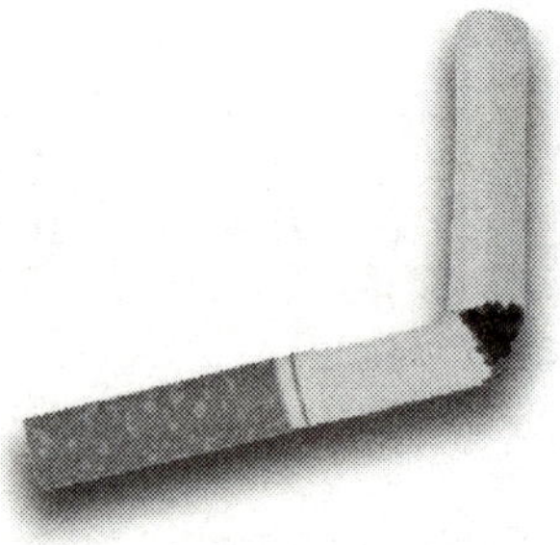

FRENCHOGRAPH

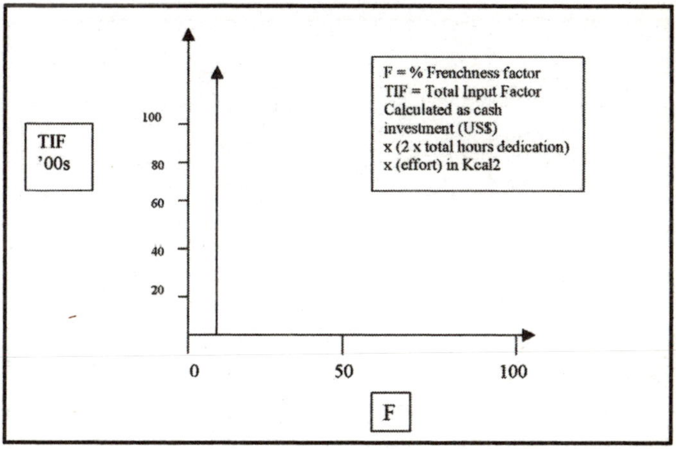

Fig. 11.1

As you can see, the total increase in overall Frenchness, even for those of us with any kind of Anglo roots (i.e. some Norman blood somewhere) is precisely zero. The inevitable result for the Japograph is, unsurprisingly, shown in scientific form thus:

JAPOGRAPH

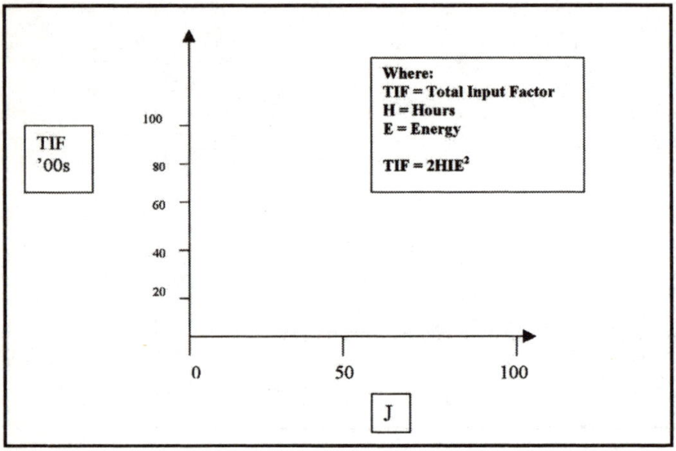

Fig. 11.2

Not particularly impressive, I'm sure you will agree. For, as we have now proved, however high factors H, I or E will go, J will always equal 0. Clearly one is never going to lose weight with that equation. Or, to put it another way, as every 40-year-old divorcee prowling around Miami's

South Beach will eventually testify, 'Wherever you go, there you are.'

But before we get too depressed about this we shall now throw ourselves a lifeline in the form of the…

ETHIOPIOGRAPH

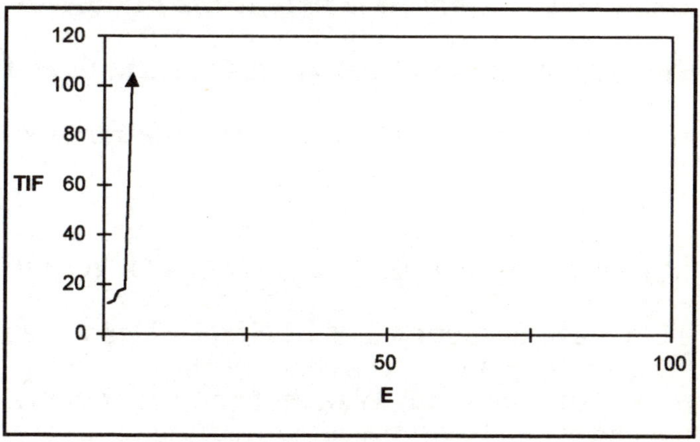

Fig. 11.3

As you can see, the main difference here is that a little bit of 'input' up the left-hand axis ACTUALLY MAKES A DIFFERENCE. And the crucial point is that you will no more get to think or feel or look like an Ethiopian than you will like a Japanese or French woman. The *only way* in which your 'E' factor percentage rating will increase is *entirely based upon your weight.* What you will *not* have here is the middle-of-the-night junk-food temptation, the extra slice of chocolate cake, the sneaky white wine spritzer.

Ethiopian women (or men) DO NOT get fat. They have no equivalent of Gérard Depardieu or Takanohana and Wakanohana, the famous sumo brothers and Japanese champion wrestlers. It is also worth noting that right now there aren't many porkers in Dafur or Rwanda either. Are you getting the pattern?

So here's how it works…

If you're *really* serious about weight loss this is one of the simplest and most effective methods. All you need to do is pick your country. You could put names in a hat or throw a dart at a map of Africa or, just trust me, Dar es Salaam will do. And that's it. Unlike many of the diets, even in this book, there is no preparation, no long drawn-out process of acclimatisation. It's easy. You're simply buying a one-way ticket to somewhere where there's virtually no food. There's no need to sell your house, sort out your bank account or cancel the milk – that will all take care of itself in time, not that it'll be any concern of yours – you're now concerned solely with a higher level of being: personal aesthetics. Just pick your day. Get out of bed, take one credit card from your purse or wallet, throw the rest over the ledge or into the street and take a train to your nearest international airport.

It is worth noting at this stage that you can eat absolutely anything you like in whatever quantities you please. In fact the real beauty of this whole plan is that this is pretty much the case throughout the whole process – it's just the actual availability of food that will decrease. No need to deal with the problems of lack of will power or giving in to temptation. Have as little willpower as you like, because pretty soon there's going to be nothing to tempt you in any way whatsoever. At the airport, simply purchase a one-way ticket to, let us say, Harare, and Bob's your uncle.

Upon arrival it may well help to buy a map of the country and identify the area with the least writing on it. Huge blank areas are always promising. All you need now is a car and a few extra cans of petrol and you're ready to become the slimmer's version of Virginia Woolf. Just point the car in your chosen direction, throw your credit card out of the window and keep driving.

And keep driving.

As long as you leave Westernised civilisation far behind there is really no wrong place to stop. The purist will tell you that you should just keep on going until you run out of fuel and go from there. And why not? It will really make no difference. The next few months can, and certainly will, take any number of unpredictable turns. The only thing of which you can be certain – as you gather, hunt or steal what you can – is that you will lose weight. No danger of weakening because, even if you do, there's no way back. It's a one-way ticket to thinness. End of story.

Madame X comments

... ***on intestinal parasites!***

The extra *joie* as far as
the Residents of War-Torn

Impoverished Territories diet is concerned is that everything you can 'gather, hunt or steal', as Dr Harlatan so elegantly puts it, is very likely to be infested with the eggs and larvae of *les parasites intensinales!*

Sans doute, you've heard of the friendly bacteria in live yoghurt and so forth that like to live in your gut. Well, you should try to think of *les parasites* as tiny dietary 'elpers too! All too often people are far too negative about having another being alive inside you! All nonsense! Remember the friend who sometimes 'elps you out with your *dîner* when you are in an expensive restaurant and you cannot eat all your food but do not want to waste it? *Alors*, try to think of *les parasites*, worms in the main, as a little bit like that kindly friend, only they are with you all the time - they will never leave you - and they help you from the inside! What could be more kindly than that?!

Let's see how it works!

In the pie next up you'll see that all the food that passes your lips is used by your body. It's very hard to lose weight this way.

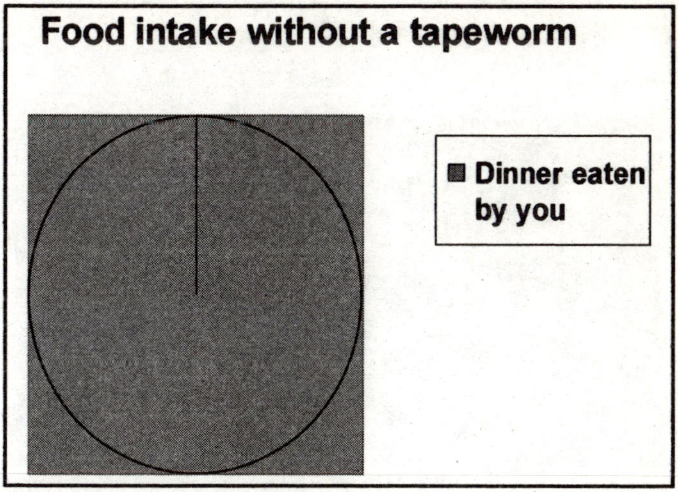

Fig. 11.4

However, just look at the next pie chart!

See how the share of food eaten by the tapeworm corresponds to a reduction in your share - even though your food *intake* hasn't actually gone down. Magic!

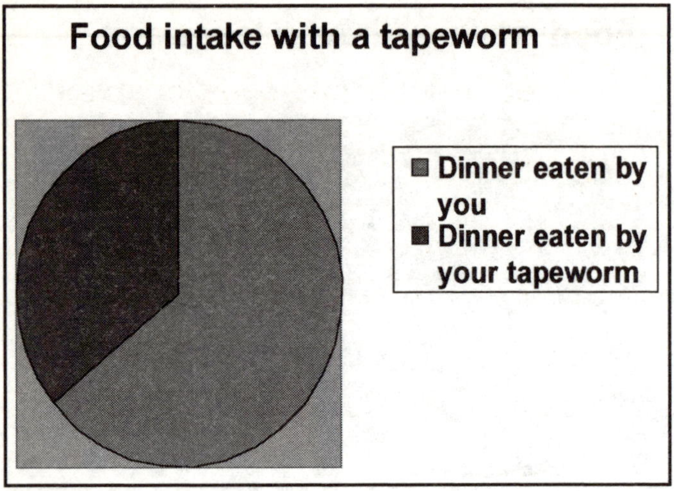

Fig 11.5

There are, in fact, many kinds of *parasite*. It is not even *nécessaire* to go to an impoverished war-torn territory, although it does help![1] *Bien sûr*, your trip to a war-torn territory will be particularly well suited to infestation, not only

[1] You might strike lucky but in Europe, for example, you could spend years eating raw meat and fish and still, unfortunately, end up wormless. Contrary to our normal advice, it is probably worth spending that little bit more to obtain food that is organic. Organic food has no chemicals that will kill off your friendly parasites.

because anything you can get hold of to eat will be *très* questionable, but also because you will be rather, how do you say it?, run down – which allows *beaucoup des occasions* for *Madame Tapeworm* and her *collègues* to get nicely settled in.

Perhaps the most *célèbre parasite* is the lovely long tapeworm, which you can find in the pork, the beef or the fish. Indeed, the tapeworm has a long and illustrious association with dieting. It is said that Victorian ladies used to take a tapeworm egg as a slimming aid and that this was a 'miracle' ingredient of some early twentieth-century diet pills too. Even the glamorous Maria Callas is associated with them. *Madame Tapeworm* helps you out with your dinner, that is for sure. *Mais aussi*, depending on which *parasite* you source, you can lose weight in other valuable ways too, including the vomiting, the diarrhoea and fidgeting, and *la mort*. Some *parasites* will even 'elp by eating *you* from the inside![2] And if you really do not think you can stomach the parasite diet, do not worry too much about it. You could use your *wimperie lamentable* to your advantage too. You might even find

[2] Operating as tiny little cosmetic surgeons e.g. hookworms.

that *thinking* about parasites helps you to lose weight.

Why do you not try the following exercise?

Step 1 Google the 'tapeworm' or the 'intestinal parasite' and 'fish'.

Step 2 Now go for a sashimi bento.

Step 3 Now think about why Japanese women do not get fat.

If you make a point of doing this at every mealtime you will see the weight drop from you! I personally have lost 10 kilos just writing this section!

Bonne chance!

DIET MIX 'N' MATCH DIET MIX 'N' MATCH DIET MIX 'N' MATCH DIET MI

You can combine this diet with...

Chain smoking and speed.

Avoid...

Narcissism and being a heartbroken man.

RESIDENTS OF WAR-TORN IMPOVERISHED TERRITORIES DON'T GET FAT

100% OF THIN PEOPLE DIE

TOP MODEL KATE ROSS'S TWENTY REASONS WHY SHE HATES THIS BOOK

1. The diets are dangerous.

2. The diets involve unsavoury lifestyle choices.

3. The hectoring tone.

4. The smugness.

5. The weird rituals.

6. The relentlessness.

6. Dr Harlatan is a charlatan.

7. Madame X is fictitious.

8. Thinness equals goodness.

9. Thinness has a morality all of its own.

10. The assumption that we all want to be thin.

11. Pity for the fat.

12. The obsession with thinness to the exclusion of all else.

13. The positive encouragement of eating disorders.

14. The dubious science.

15. The diets involve sustaining serious medical conditions.

16. The cultural chauvinism.

17. The spurious reductionism.

18. The cashing-in on a trend.

20. It's morally wrong, dammit, not like those other diet books!

APPENDIX 1

[FILL IN YOURSELF] DON'T GET FAT

Design your own MQ diet!

Go on! It's easy and fun too. All you have to do is follow the form of Madame X and myself.

1. Think of a type of person who normally ends up rather thin.

2. Think of some (but by no means all) of the things that person does. (N.B. They don't necessarily need to be

things done to try and get thin.) Let's call them lifestyle aspects.

3. Choose which lifestyle aspects you want to link to the end result (i.e. thinness). Don't worry if the link seems very spurious. Madame X and I have found that this really doesn't matter at all...

4. And you're away! We've drawn you up a template diet plan. All you need do is fill it in!

To get you started

Talk, briefly here about how rubbish all other diets are... and how only the untapped secrets of your miracle-plan have any hope of lasting success...

How it works

Explain briefly how your diet works here:

Show how it works in a graph (label axis and plotted line).

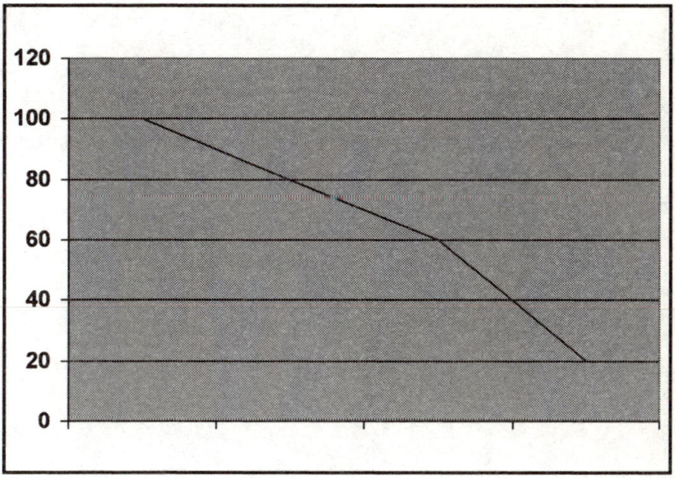

Support the graph with notes and explanations of abbreviations – or not (your choice).

Blather on a bit more here:

Scientific diagram here:

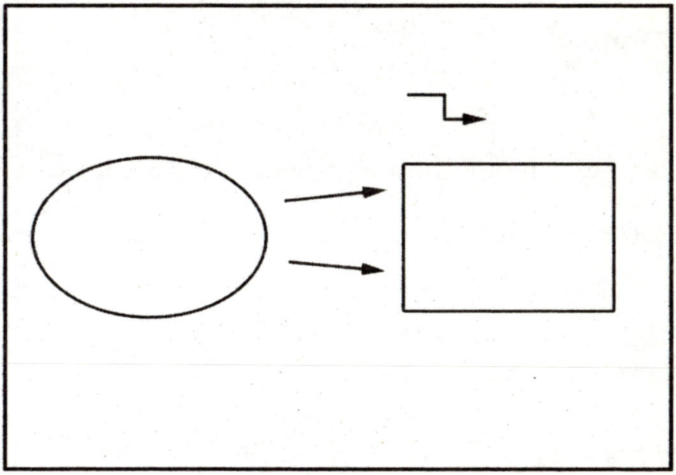

Again, support the graph with notes and explanations of abbreviations – only if you feel like it.

Your 7-Day Miracle Plan

Monday

Suggest any method which equates to not eating too much here:

Tuesday

Make a variation on Monday:

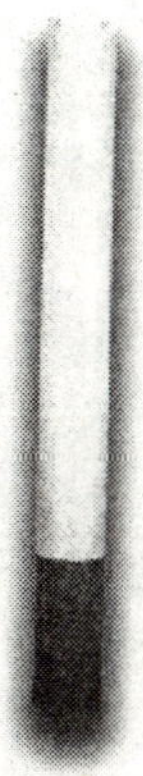

Wednesday

I think you'll be getting the idea now...

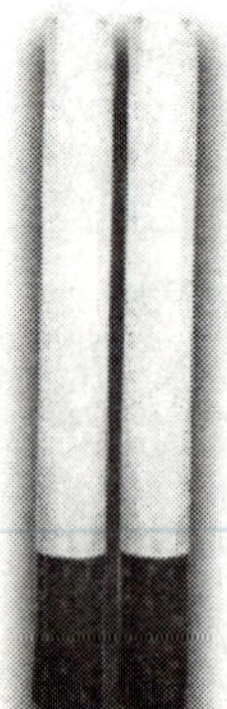

Thursday

Try to be a little more adventurous with your diet recommendations for today; mid-week is boring and tough.

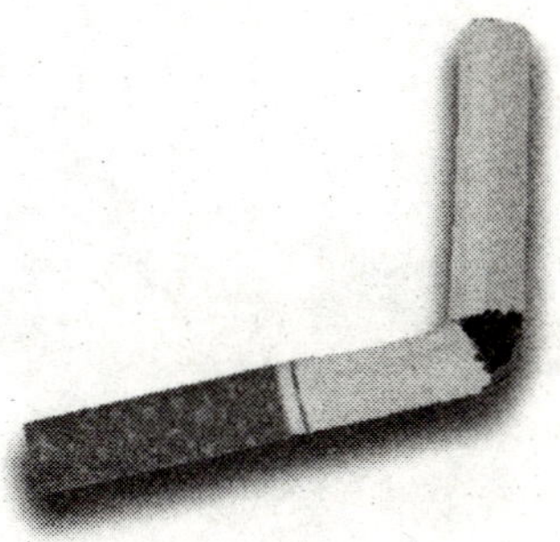

Friday

By now the days should be beginning to blur into one, so keep the pressure up.

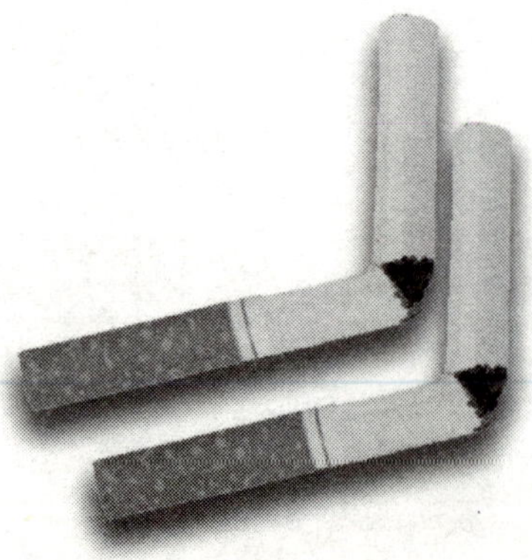

Saturday

Rack it up now.

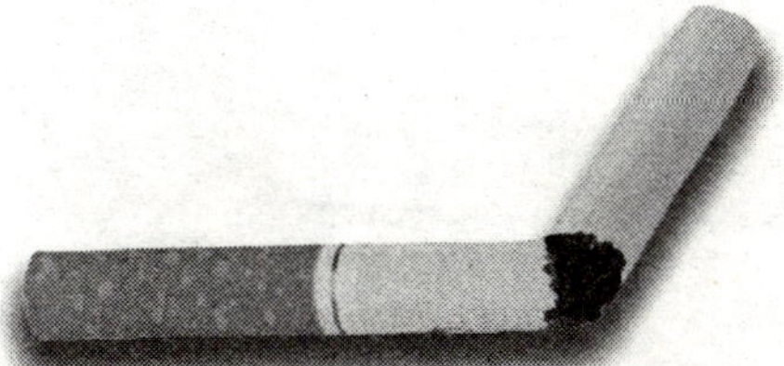

Sunday

Similar to the rest of the week but introduce a treat that no right-thinking person would ever consider to be a treat:

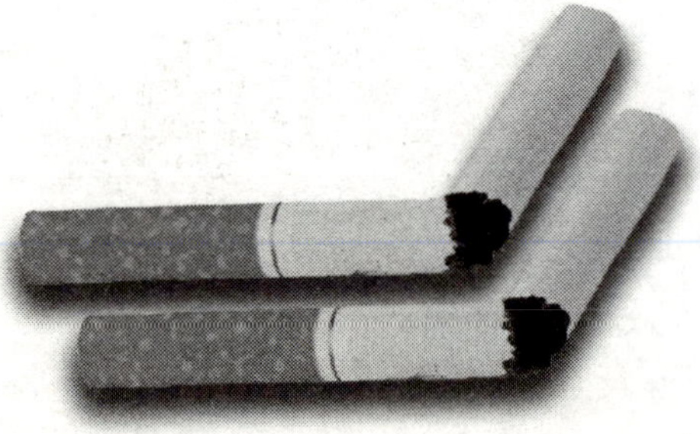

And that's it. It really is that simple! Go on, write your diet book today! There's no need to be shy now that you know that any old bollocks will do.

Where would we be without Madame X commenting on your diet?

C'est merveilleux, etc.

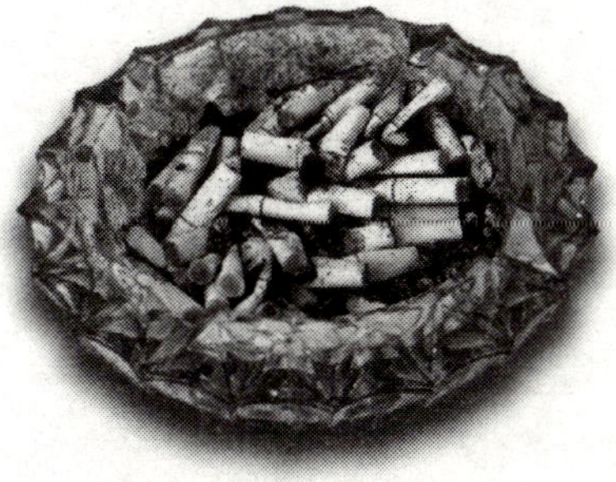

DIET MIX 'N' MATCH DIET MIX 'N' MATCH DIET MIX 'N' MATCH DIET MI

You can combine this diet with...

Avoid...

ABOUT THE AUTHORS

MADAME X

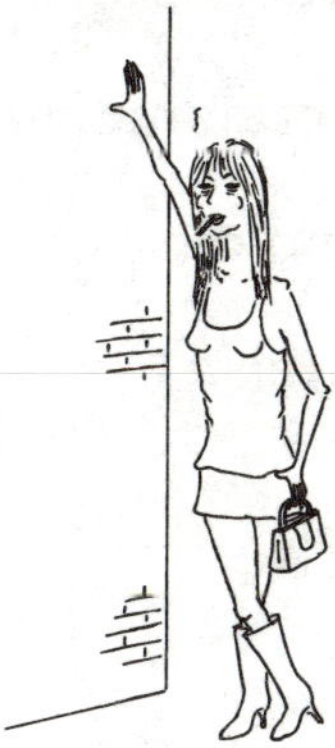

Madame X is a smoking, drinking, substance-abusing, surprisingly well-read crack whore.

DR C HARLATAN

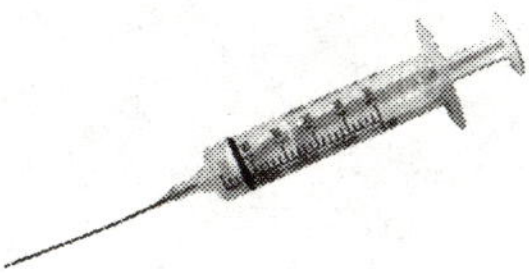

Dr C Harlatan is not a doctor.

Go to www.smackheadsdontgetfat.com for your downloadable New Labour Moralometer Wall Chart and questionnaire to find out how morally questionable you are!

All Crombie Jardine books are available from High Street bookshops, Amazon, Littlehampton Book Services, or Bookpost P.O.Box 29, Douglas, Isle of Man, IM99 1BQ. Tel: 01624 677 237 email: bookshop@enterprise.net (free postage and packing within the UK).

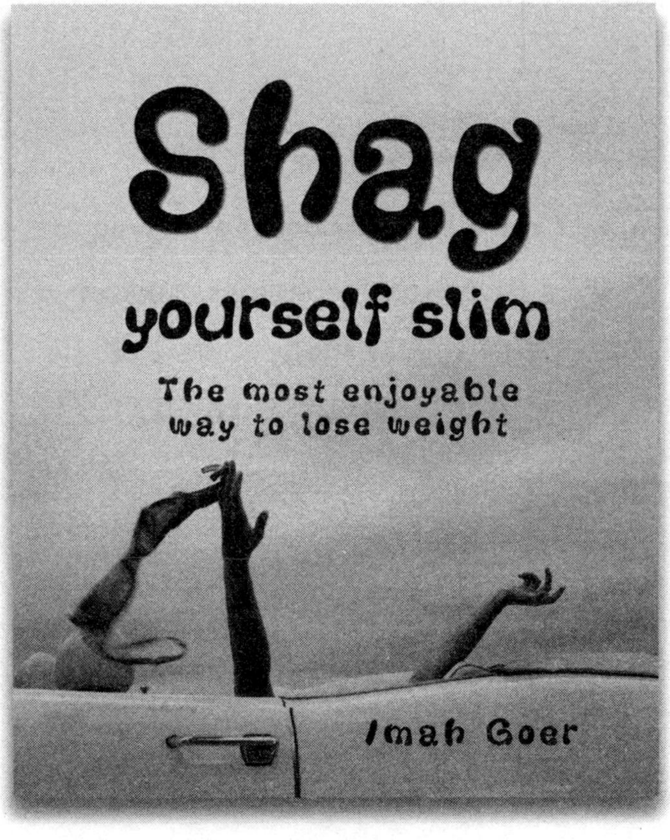

ISBN 1-905102-03-8

£2.99

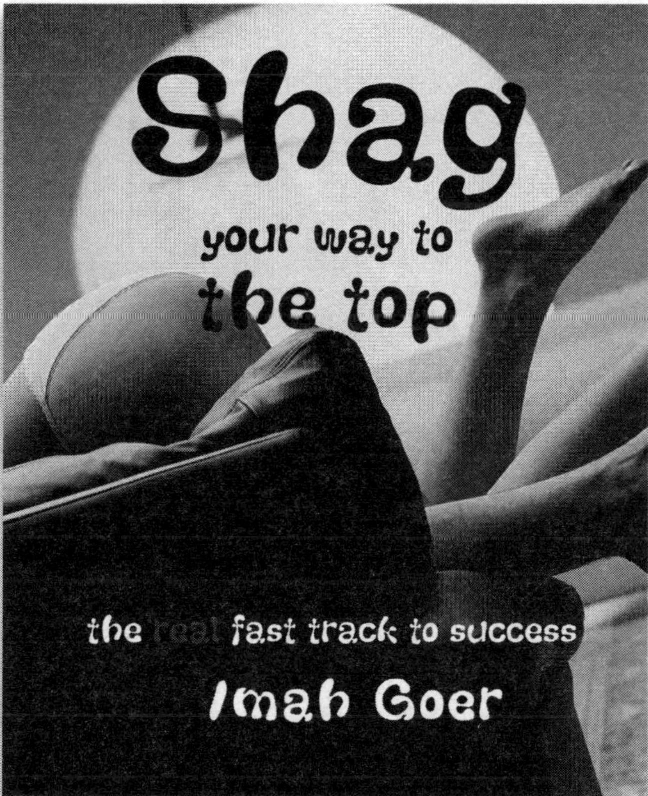

ISBN 1-905102-17-8

£2.99